ONE WEEK LOAN

Youth and social policy
Youth citizenship and young careers

Bob Coles
University of York

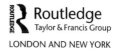

Routledge
Taylor & Francis Group

LONDON AND NEW YORK

First published in 1995 by Routledge
2 Park Square, Milton Park, Abingdon, Oxon, OX14 4RN
270 Madison Ave, New York NY 10016

Transferred to Digital Printing 2008

British Library Cataloguing-in-Publication Data
A catalogue record for this book is available from the British Library.

Library of Congress Cataloging-in-Publication Data
Coles, Bob.
    Youth and social policy : youth citizenship and young careers /
Bob Coles.
        p.   cm.
    Includes bibliographical references and index.
    ISBN 1-85728-303-1 (hc.) — ISBN 1-85728-304-X (pbk.)
    1. Youth—Government policy. I. Title.
HQ796.C644 1995
305.23'5—dc   95-16039
                                                                CIP

ISBN: 1-85728-303-1 HB
          1-85728-304-X PB

Typeset in Sabon and Gill Sans.

Publisher's Note
The publisher has gone to great lengths to ensure the quality of this
reprint but points out that some imperfections in the original
may be apparent.

For Chris and Jo and all people of their generation who were in
so many different ways the subject of, and subjected to, this book

Contents

Acknowledgements

When I first planned to write this book I thought I already had it in my head. How wrong I was. I knew what I wanted the book to cover but having a grasp of the material in order to do so, and to do so coherently and in a manner which made it accessible to students, was another matter. As I prepared to write each chapter I experienced the panic of someone who was setting themselves up as an expert without a thorough grasp of the literature which would justify the project. In writing this book I have drawn upon the knowledge and wisdom of many people at the University of York and elsewhere. To all who have helped I record a very special thanks.

The bulk of the book was written during a research term. Many encouraged me to spend it away from York but I resisted, sometimes to my cost, but mostly to the benefit of the book. The rich array of social policy talent at York did come up with the goods in terms of always seeming to have experts on hand when I most needed them – to beg, steal and borrow books, research reports and ideas. I called on so many people in the Department of Social Policy and Social Work and its associated research units, institutes and centres that it seems invidious to name specific individuals. But I must thank Karl Atkin, Sally Baldwin, Michael Hirst and Julie Seymour for feeding me material on young people with disabilities; Debbi Baldwin, Leslie Hicks and Ian Sinclair for material and ideas on young people in care; Jonathan Bradshaw for material on young people and the family; Carol-Ann Hooper for guiding me to the inner mysteries of the Children Act, 1989: Tina Davis for guidance on social security and benefits; and Steve Craine and Tony Fowles for material on crime and the criminal justice system. Outside York, Pat Ainley, David Ashton and Phil Brown made very helpful comments on my initial ideas. Gill Robson helped plumb me into to the rich seam of data from the Youth Cohort Studies. Gill Jones kindly read and commented on several chapters and kept me supplied with details of her own research much of which proved of critical importance at the right time. Graduate and undergraduate students also helped shape my ideas especially members of the Thursday night Youth Policy reading group (Debbi Baldwin, Stewart Kirk, Lynn Robinson, Elizabeth Storrs and Jon Tan) all of whom made useful comments on early draft chapters to which they were subjected. None of these are to blame for the finished product, but helped me move from chronic ignorance to the confidence to put things down on paper and finally turn them into print.

Much of the book is about young people, family relationships and the traumas of youth transitions. I was acutely aware as I was writing some of the chapters that I was writing about me and us as well as they and them. To Mary Maynard I owe so many debts of intellectual and social companionship such that the book would still be an idle twinkle in my imagination without her help. As always, she has kept me going through the dark hours, tolerated my obsessiveness, and corrected the worst features of a writer who still bears the scars of an 11+ failure with only a fleeting grasp of the rules of spelling and grammar. Chris and Jo helped too in their own sweet ways as they wrestled with the problems of youth transitions whilst their father merely wrote about them and did so whilst being parsimonious with his parental time. They variously helped me to be mousified, windowed, adequately competent with the technology of the late twentieth century, tolerantly supportive of my Peter Pan greying obsession with youth, and surprised me even further by seeming interested in some of what I wrote.

This book is about Youth and Social Policy but it is intended to stimulate a more informed, comprehensive and sensitised policy agenda for youth. It is an attempt to bring to the attention of social scientists the circumstances of many young people who are often ignored in the mainstream literature. It is they for whom the book is written. They deserve my thanks for being my continued inspiration But they all deserve our better knowledge, research. concern and attention as we plan for the future welfare of all young people.

Chapter One

Youth, youth transitions and social policy

This book is about youth and social policy and as such it will outline some of the major problems being faced by young people in contemporary Britain and highlight what policy makers could, and should, do to help. It is a theoretical as well as an empirical book in that it attempts both to develop a theoretical framework for a social policy of youth and to describe the ways in which the condition of youth has been substantially transformed in the last quarter of the twentieth century. As we shall see, youth policy in Britain has developed in a largely piecemeal and uncoordinated way, with each different Department of State addressing only those aspects of "youth problems" which it sees as falling within its domain. To counteract this, some writers have called for a Minister for Youth to co-ordinate better the disparate activities of various arms of government (Coleman & Warren-Adamson 1992), while others have argued for a more holistic approach to the study of youth to be made by academic researchers, policy makers and practitioners (Jones & Wallace 1992). The academic study of youth certainly has mirrored state policy in its uncoordinated and "atomistic" approach, with separate branches of the social sciences focusing on different facets of young people's lives. The problems of adolescence have received most attention in psychology (Coleman & Hendry 1992, Hendry 1983, Noller & Callan 1991), while social work has focused on the issue of child protection and caring for children (Fox-Harding 1991, Parton 1991). The social inequalities of educational attainment and the problems of transition from school to work have dominated the interests of sociologists of education (Brown 1987, Gleeson 1989, Raffe 1988). Since the 1980s, labour market scholars and youth specialists have concentrated their attention on a shrinking youth labour market, the growth of youth unemployment and the impact of a plethora of training schemes on young "careers" (Ainley 1990, Coles 1988, Finn 1987, Gleeson 1989, Hollands 1990, Lee et al. 1990, Wallace & Cross 1990) while delinquency, hooliganism, deviance and young offenders have figured prominently in criminology (Becker 1963, Little 1990, Marsh et al. 1978, Muncie 1984, Parker et al. 1981). In the 1970s, sociologists of youth focused their attention on the development of youth subcultures and distinctive youth life styles (Brake 1980, Hall & Jefferson 1976, Hebdige 1979). More recently, others have addressed the more specific issues of youth suicides, changes in sexual behaviour, drug and alcohol abuse and the threat of HIV/AIDS (Aggleton et al. 1991, Brannen et al. 1994, Plant & Plant 1992, Woodroffe et al. 1993). Many of these themes will be brought together in the pages of this book.

The first five chapters will examine the concepts of career and citizenship and will explore how the application of these concepts to the lives of young people can aid our understanding of their needs, rights and interests, and better focus attention on the impact of social policy on young people's welfare. The book will, however, pay particular regard to some groups of young people who have been excluded from most sociological texts on youth, and Chapters 6–8 will focus attention on the special problems of particularly vulnerable sections of youth: young people in local authority care; young people with disabilities and with special needs; and young people involved in crime. This book is intended to be much more than just factual in its attempts to break new ground by developing a theoretical framework for our understanding of youth and social policy. Before moving on to discuss the main theoretical concepts which will act as a framework for our analysis, it is, perhaps, important to attempt to define "youth" and the aspects of social policy covered here.

Social policy and the study of youth

It is important to start with some preliminary definitions of what we mean by "youth" and "social policy", even though such definitions cannot be simple or straightforward. Compared to the nebulous concept of youth, social policy is relatively easy to define. It is the study of welfare and welfare systems and the ways in which systems of welfare do, or do not, meet human needs. The discipline of social policy is an applied social science drawing upon sociology, politics, economics, history and demography in addressing issues of welfare. It grew out of the study of social administration which was, arguably, a more descriptive discipline in examining how the various institutions of welfare were organized and administered (UGC 1989). The distinctive perspective of social policy was developed as a means of giving the study of social administration both an evaluative stance and a greater critical potential. Students of social policy are thus expected both to understand the structures of welfare provision and to be able to examine how such structures can be better directed towards meeting needs.

Some studies in social policy concentrate upon institutional provision (Young 1985, Hills 1991) and, following this tradition, this book will examine some of the key institutional areas affecting young people: education, training and the labour market; housing, health and social security; institutions of care; crime and the penal system. Other aspects of social policy focus upon particular client groups: people with disabilities; the homeless; the elderly (Barnes 1991, Biggs 1993, Swain et al. 1993, Thornton 1990). Such studies help us to examine how sets of welfare institutions together do, or do not, serve the best interests of specific client groups who are sometimes argued to have distinctive types of welfare need (Glendinning & Millar 1987). Social policy also often focuses attention on the most vulnerable sections of the community and the ones who most require the help of state agencies in both supporting them and protecting their welfare. Such studies examine the co-ordination (or lack of co-ordination) of welfare institutions, gaps in welfare provision, and the plight of those who appear to slip through the nets of welfare systems (Barnes 1991, Thornton 1990). In focusing on the most vulnerable, this book does not seek to mark these groups out as necessarily different or pathological. Rather, it will be argued, it is by concentrating attention upon the most vulnerable groups, that we may be better able to understand the needs of all young people.

What is meant by "youth"?

We must also be clear about what we mean by "youth" and why young people constitute a distinctive group. This book will maintain the distinction between "youth", which will be used to denote a phase in the life course, and young people, the group who are at this phase in the life course. At its simplest, youth can be defined as an interstitial phase in the life course between childhood and adulthood (Jones & Wallace 1992). Such a definition, of course, begs the questions as to what we mean by childhood and adulthood, and when one ends and the other begins. Furthermore, these are almost impossible to answer in any categorical way. As Jones & Wallace argue, such statuses are constantly in flux and subject to complex processes of negotiation and renegotiation "between young people and their families, their peers and the institutions of the wider society" (Jones & Wallace 1992: 4). These are, as we will see, the key actors in the social construction and reconstruction of the statuses of youth. But, if we examine the ways in which welfare systems are differentially designed for children and adults we can discern some stark contrasts. Welfare systems designed for children are organized so as to offer opportunities and support for their physical, emotional, social, moral and educational development and to protect them from abuse and exploitation (Coleman & Warren-Adamson 1992, Franklin 1986). Some of this is done indirectly through support for the family, but it also occurs through the direct provision of services for children and young people by agencies of the state. As we shall see in later chapters, welfare policy accepts that "childhood" has a status of "dependency". In many societies, and for most children, this dependency is largely provided for within the household and the family. Children are expected to be looked after by their families and to be economically dependent upon them. Many welfare systems offer economic and social support to parents with children, together with state support for children who fall outside biological families, because of bereavement or because such families cannot cope adequately with the upbringing. In circumstances such as these, where children are for some reason detached from their biological families, children are offered surrogate families through fostering, adoption, or places in special institutions, such as children's homes (Gottesmann 1994). In Britain and elsewhere, children are also provided with welfare services beyond the confines of the family, through schools, nurseries, medical care and other services based in the community. Where children or young people are regarded as severely disturbed, violent, or potentially "at risk", they may be catered for in specially designed "secure accommodation" provided for or paid for by agencies of the state. Children and young people up to the age of 16 are obliged to be educated and to attend school, and legally their parents, or guardians, must ensure that they do so. In most developed welfare systems children are also protected by law from various forms of exploitation. In Britain, children cannot legally engage in sexual activity, and cannot marry or vote (Jones & Wallace 1992). Nor can they take up many forms of paid employment until a specific age, and then only in limited and controlled circumstances. Children cannot enter into legal contracts or legally own property until the age of majority of 18 in England and Wales, though they can at the age of 16 in Scotland (Jones 1994). Parents are legally responsible for making certain that children are properly cared for, looked after and fulfil all their legal obligations. If children commit criminal offences they are dealt with by special courts, and their parents (as well as the children themselves) can be called upon to answer for their actions, blamed for not exercising proper care and control, and in some cases share in any reparation required by the courts (Ashworth et al. 1992). Children are, therefore, deemed to be dependent upon adult society, are protected from exploitation by adult society, and are nurtured and provided for by both the family and the state. The family is regarded as a natural haven in which protection and dependence can be achieved, but the state acts as guarantor for the welfare and development of all children.

Adults, on the other hand, are accorded different rights and responsibilities. They can marry, vote and enter into contracts, and they are held responsible for their own actions in both the civil and criminal courts. By and large they are expected to provide for their own economic means of support, to engage in paid work, to provide themselves with a living, and to pay taxes towards the cost of general welfare services and the social security of others (Marshall 1981). Some adults who cannot find paid work, or who are beyond the age of retirement, receive state support through various forms of social security, unless they are female and living in households, in which case they may be deemed to be financially dependent upon another male wage earner (Lister 1991). In short, adults are treated as full "citizens" and as such are regarded as independent and responsible human beings. A more detailed discussion of all these issues will be made when considering the concept of citizenship in Chapters 4 and 5, but for the moment it is sufficient to recognize that differences in age-status result in different patterns of rights and responsibilities.

Young people are treated neither as children nor as adults. As will be seen in Chapter 4, under the Children Act 1989, they are considered to be capable of making some decisions about their own futures, but are also considered to need both some protection from exploitation and abuse, and some help and guidance in making wise decisions about their own welfare and careers. They are thus regarded, in part, as both independent choice-making human beings, but also as dependent upon other people (and especially their parents) for care, guidance and support. The full rights and responsibilities of adulthood are given gradually, and at different ages, while parents and legal guardians are expected and required to help young people make the transition to full adult status (Jones & Wallace 1992). Legally, the rights and responsibilities of youth and adulthood present a complex (if not chaotic) picture of the transition to adulthood. In England and Wales, young people can: be at least in part held "responsible" for crime at the age of 10; undertake part-time employment (between 7am and 7pm) after the age of 13; be liable to pay full fare on public transport (buses and trains) at the age of 14; cease to attend full-time education at 16 and legally engage in heterosexual sex with consent at the same age; vote, be sent to an adult prison, be required to undergo national service and marry without parental consent after the "age of majority" at 18; until 1994, not legally engage in male homosexual activities until the age of 21 (reduced to the age of 18 in 1994); and not receive social security at an adult rate, in the form of income support if they are unemployed, until the age of 25 (Craig 1991, Wright 1988). When they are in the care of local authorities rather than their parents', young people's views must be taken into account in deciding where and with whom they should live, and they may be supported by their local authorities up to the age of 21. If they are homeless and under the age of 16, local authorities must arrange accommodation for them, but after that age, housing may be provided only if they are thought to be vulnerable or at risk (Anderson et al. 1993, Thornton 1990, White et al. 1990). These and other legal rights help to illustrate that, in legal terms, there is no clear end to the status of childhood and no clear age at which young people are given full adult rights and responsibilities. In short, the legal definitions of childhood, youth and adulthood present a complex array of definitions which have been developed by the different institutions of the state, for different purposes, and at different moments in history. Such definitions certainly do not aid any clear chronological definition of youth.

Many rights and responsibilities are, furthermore, dependent not only upon chronological age, but upon participation in some social institution. In this sense, young people's rights are status contingent. So, while young people are entitled by law to finish full-time education at the age of 16, they are also given entitlements to "free" tertiary education and training between the ages of 16 and 18 and local authority grants and loans to support the continuation of their education. While they are in full-time education, young people are expected to be financially dependent upon their parents, and while some grants and loans are given by the state towards their maintenance, such grants are "means tested" and, as such, are dependent upon the assessed income of parents. While in full-time education, young people may be entitled to free medical treatment (up to the age of 19), and special discounted prices on public transport through student and young people's "rail cards", further evidence that some rights are dependent upon status rather than chronological age. This complex catalogue of "rights" suggests that young people are granted a status of both semi-dependency and semi-independency. Society, it seems, recognizes that young people should be accorded some rights and responsibilities in decision making about their future, and some support and guidance in doing so. Careers officers are especially committed to the giving of guidance and advice directly to young people, often deliberately excluding their parents from the guidance process (Coles 1991). Yet young people are still assumed to be largely dependent upon their parents, especially in an economic sense. Youth is thus a period of transition from childhood to adulthood which has neither a clear chronological beginning nor end. Some rights and responsibilities (such as the legal right to engage in part-time employment) are given as early as 13, even though, as we will see in Chapter 2, the law is widely ignored. Others, such as full rights to adult income support, are delayed until the age of 25 (Harris 1989). Furthermore, these rights and entitlements have been subject to change as the social and economic circumstances of young people have changed. In the United Kingdom, rights to Income Support for 16–18-year-olds were withdrawn in 1988 because the government expected that all young people should either be in full-time education or undertaking Youth Training (Craig 1991, Harris 1989). The same Social Security Act which brought about these changes also introduced a special youth rate for 18–25-year-olds on the assumption that young people would still be living within the households of their parents and, thus, experience a lower cost of living (Harris 1989). The legal definitions of youth dependency are, therefore, contingent upon other social and economic factors and assumptions.

Youth as a series of transitions

Rather than seek a complex and often unsatisfactory age definition for youth, many academic writers have defined it as a series of transitions (Banks et al. 1992, Jones & Wallace 1992). Achieving the status of adulthood is thus dependent upon successfully making at least some of these transitions, rather than reaching some arbitrary chronological age. The main transitions of youth which are of critical importance are as follows:

 – the transition from full-time education and training to a full-time job in the labour market (the school-to-work transition)
 – the transition from family of origin (mainly the biological family) to family of destination (the domestic transition)
 – the transition from residence with parents (or surrogate parents) to living away from them (the housing transition).

One of the main concepts used within this book to theorize these transitions is the concept of "career". By career is meant the sequence of statuses through which young people pass as they move from childhood dependency to adulthood. Some of these statuses may be prescribed by law, some will be the result of the intervention of an "agency" of the state, while others will be "chosen" by young people themselves, although often under the strong influence of their parents. But whatever the basis on which a particular status is allocated, this status sets in train a series of social processes which has the potentiality to "determine" the likely course of a young person's future status sequence. Under the age of 16, all young people within the United Kingdom are required to be in full-time education. The particular school they attend and the type of education they experience are the result of a series of decisions made by educational authorities about the provision of educational establishments and what the authorities and/or their parents deem to be appropriate for the educational development of each child. Parents are often involved in a key role in determining what they think is appropriate for their children, but in the case of children and young people being considered "vulnerable" or "at risk", social workers and social service departments may also be involved in the decision-making process. Partly on the basis of an assessment of a young person's needs, and partly based upon the wishes of parents, a young person may experience full-time education in a variety of different institutions, from neighbourhood comprehensive schools, to private (boarding or non-boarding) schools, to special schools (designed to educate those with special educational needs), to children's homes (with or without special educational provision), to Youth Treatment Centres designed to cope with highly disturbed young people in a secure setting. In later chapters of this book we will outline the ways in which the decisions to allocate this "status" to young people at this early stage in their career carry with them long-term consequences for future career development.

The concept of "career" as a series of staged status sequences is important in that each step in the sequence can be shown to determine future steps. It should be emphasized straight away that the notion of "determination" is not being used here in a strong, precise or mathematical sense. It is not being argued that one stage automatically leads to the next but, rather, that the attainment of each status position, in turn, has the capacity both to open up and close down future opportunities. Thus, for instance, attaining educational qualifications at the age of 16 may open up the possibility of further full-time tertiary education between the ages of 16 and 18, and further qualifications gained at 18 may, in turn, open up the possibility of full-time higher education for three or more years. Good academic qualifications may thus enhance the possibility of a longer career in education. They may also serve to delay entry into the labour market until many young people reach their early 20s. This status sequence of an extended post-16 educational career does not, of course, follow automatically from attaining good qualifications at the age of 16. Some young people with equally good qualifications may "choose" to enter the labour market at the age of 16 or 18. But without attaining the requisite number of qualifications, a young person may have little alternative but to leave school at 16 and seek work in the labour market. On the other hand, as we will see in Chapters 5–8, should the decision be made that a young person should receive pre-16 education at a special school, in a children's home, or in a Youth Treatment Centre, this often has grave consequences for the likelihood of their attaining the requisite levels of qualifications at the age of 16 which would allow them to pursue either an advanced course of education after that age or a training place with good employment prospects. For these young people, the decision to allocate a particular educational status before the age of 16 sets severe limits to the post-16 careers likely to be open to them.

For those who are successful in gaining good qualifications at the ages of 16 and 18, obtaining a place in higher education may also offer further opportunities for them to move away from their parental home and so develop a "housing career" (Jones 1987). Alternatively, getting a (good) job and earning a wage may give people the financial means to leave home and/or set up a new home with a partner or spouse. Young people who enter the labour market before the age of 20 are much more likely to marry earlier than those who go on to higher education, so decisions made about a career in education are likely to have an impact upon their domestic careers. Those who develop "extended transitions" through education are more likely to delay their "domestic careers" (Jones 1987). Those who experience "fractured transitions", through being unemployed for extended periods, are also likely to suspend decisions to marry or start a family (Wallace 1987). Each of the three main transitions do, therefore, interrelate and the status gained in one may both "determine" and "be determined by" the status sequences which are likely to be attained in another.

The three main transition lines described above contain structures of opportunities for young people. So far, they have been presented only as a series of structured choices which, before the age of 16, are made either by young people and their parents, or by other agencies responsible for young people's welfare. At the age of 16+ a young person may "choose" whether to stay on at school, go on to sixth-form studies or take courses in colleges of further education, take part in youth training or seek employment. Yet these main structures of choice are themselves determined by social and economic conditions and these, in turn, are largely shaped by social and economic policies. Policy developments can and do extend, restrict or reframe the opportunity structures available to young people and we will examine these developments in Chapters 2 and 3. Well-qualified 16- or 18-year-olds may formally have the opportunity to continue with their education, but their real opportunities to do so may depend on the number of places available at college or university and the willingness and capabilities of either the state or their parents to meet the costs of supporting them when they are there. Both education policy and the resources of the parent generation can, therefore, influence the real nature of opportunity structures. Educational and labour market careers are thus influenced not only by the qualifications attained by young people, or by their individual career choices alone, but also by state policies. Public expenditure on such things as education and training, and the buoyancy of the economy, all impact upon the choice process. Young people may have the legal right to leave full-time education at the age of 16 and enter the labour market, but their chances of gaining employment are dependent upon employers having jobs they are willing to offer them. Thus labour market conditions, too, fundamentally affect choice patterns. If there are few jobs available in the local labour market, or if they are perceived by young people as being of limited long-term value to their career development, they may "choose" not to enter the labour market and continue with their education.

Similarly, moving into independent accommodation is dependent not only on choice, preference and access to resources, but also upon the state of the housing market, including the provision of accommodation for students, trainees and workers wishing to study, train and work away from home (Jones 1993a). Youth transitions must, therefore, be examined from the point of view of both the choice patterns of young people and the ways in which economic and social policies help to shape opportunity structures. The interplay of each side of this equation produces the "social structuration" of youth (Bryant & Jary 1991, Giddens 1979, Giddens 1991). This term, developed by Giddens, implies that we must take account of both social and economic institutions which determine structures of opportunity and the agency of young people in "choosing" a particular "career" option.

Youth "trajectories" and the reproduction of "difference"

There has been some debate in the recent sociological literature on youth as to how far young people's "careers" may be said to be "determined" by the social and economic conditions in which they are brought up (Banks et al. 1992, Bates & Riseborough 1993, Furlong 1992). Some authors prefer to use the term "trajectory" rather than "career" to emphasize the force of circumstances in "determining" the likelihood that particular status sequences will be followed. Roberts, for example, remains a firm believer in the notion of "trajectory" – "the connotation of young people being somehow propelled along awaiting channels towards predetermined destinations" (Bates & Riseborough 1993: 229). Sociological interest in examining the three main transitions has also helped to focus attention upon the ways in which these also seem to aid the reproduction of social structural advantage and disadvantage. Four main dimensions of difference and disadvantage have most commonly been identified:

- social class background
- sex-gender
- locality
- ethnicity.

Until the mid-1980s most studies had concentrated on the impact of social class background on those attempting the school-to-work transition (Ashton & Field 1976, Brown 1987, Furlong 1992, Jenkins 1983, Willis 1977). The mid-1980s saw the publication of a number of studies which recognized the importance of both gender and locality in mediating the impact of class (Ashton et al. 1986, Coles 1988, Griffin 1985, Raffe 1988, Skeggs 1986, 1990). During the second half of the 1980s, the Economic and Social Research Council (ESRC) funded a major research initiative on the lives of young people known as the ESRC 16–19 Initiative (Banks et al. 1992). This project attempted to describe and "map" youth transitions between the end of compulsory full-time education and entry into the labour market, as these occurred in the late 1980s. In trying to conceptualize even this single transition process, the researchers had some difficulty. The main report largely follows the balancing of "structuration" and "agency" as outlined above. It defines youth as "the time when critical *choices* are made" (Banks et al. 1992: 1, emphasis added). Yet it also simultaneously recognizes that, in making these choices, "a young person is subject to 'structural' influences stemming from the social and cultural groups to which he or she belongs. Thus social class, gender, and ethnicity will all play a part in shaping aspirations, as do characteristics of the locality in which the young person lives" (Banks et al. 1992: 1–2). The main report further recognizes that these influences are "mediated" through informal networks of social relationships involving parents, friends and peer groups, as well as the more formal networks of advice and guidance provided by teachers and careers advisers. This distinction is also made by Killeen in examining the impact of the two different types of networks on the decisions young people make about their post-16 career options (Killeen et al. 1992).

Concentration on the analysis of "trajectory", however, runs the danger of de-emphasizing choice and focusing attention on social structural determinacy. So, for example, although Roberts recognizes that there are, in the 1990s, a myriad of different academic and vocational courses in post-16 education, and a range of different jobs and Youth Training places, he argues that there are really only three main "trajectories": successful trajectories leading to good jobs, less successful trajectories leading to respectable working-class jobs, and trajectories resulting in insecure employment, training and bouts of unemployment (Roberts 1993). Despite there being a growing number of "options" available to young people between the ages of 16 and 18, the expansion of "choice" in post-16 education and training he regards as being only a "mirage" of social change and, as such, largely an illusionary and cosmetic expansion. He argues that the various routes and trajectories through education and training to employment pass through three main phases: pre-16 education; education, training and work between the ages of 16 and 18; and post-18 careers. The first and critical phase is prior to the age of 16, when young people's abilities and aptitudes in education lead eventually to either good, bad or indifferent 16+ qualifications. He regards the type of qualification level they achieve at 16+ as being critical in "determining" what happens afterwards. He further regards the qualification band they achieve at 16+ as evidence of the way in which they were "already partly programmed" to be "propelled along awaiting career routes". For the most successful young people, good qualifications act as a passport into the second phase (between the ages of 16 and 18), in which the educationally successful gain access to the most secure routes. The status sequence may be either through further academic education, employer-led training or skilled employment. Whichever "path" is followed, good qualifications at the age of 16 correlate with a "successful outcome" thereafter. The less successful, in terms of qualifications, here split into two different trajectories. The fortunate secure either "good jobs" (but not "top jobs" – be they "manual" or "white-collar" sectors of the labour market), or places in youth training which are both employer led and likely to lead to employment afterwards. They thus attain the same "respectable working-class" jobs as those who left school for such jobs at the age of 16 in the 1970s (Willis 1977, Brown 1987). The less fortunate group, often with few or poor qualifications at the age of 16, leave school only to gain insecure and low-paid jobs, or places on Youth Training which are highly unlikely to lead to secure employment at 18. Those propelled along this "trajectory" are highly likely to experience a mixture of low-paid, insecure employment, temporary places on other low-grade training schemes, and bouts of unemployment. Some of this third group thus become trapped in what Craine has called the "black magic roundabout" of training schemes, unemployment and yet more training schemes. They become more disillusioned and detached from any real prospect of secure employment as they are conscripted into an endless cycle of schemes for the unemployed and some at least become tempted by alternative (and non-legal) means of making a living (Craine 1994, MacDonald 1994). Others have referred to this group as experiencing "fractured transitions" (Jones & Wallace 1992, Willis 1984). We will review the evidence about the development of extended and fractured transitions in the next two chapters. What concerns us here is the conceptualization of youth transitions.

The reason Roberts regards youth transitions as "trajectories" is that he claims that the routes young people follow are largely determined by social class and locality. Young people from middle-class families in the ESRC 16–19 Initiative study were twice as likely to find themselves on the "successful trajectory" than those from working-class families. Seventy per cent of them were destined for success. On the other hand, he claims that two-thirds of those from working-class families experienced "failure" at one or more of the three-stage status transitions he describes. The majority of the teenagers covered by the

ESRC studies were not, as Roberts points out, free to make strategic choices about how best to secure stable employment, nor "free to roam throughout the national labour market" (Bates & Riseborough 1993: 231). Apart from those in private education or with private means of geographical mobility, they were constrained by the localities in which they lived (MacDonald 1988). Significantly, the ESRC studies also ignored those who escape local conditions, through entry into the military services or into occupations or training programmes such as nursing or catering, which some studies have shown to be of some importance as escape routes from collapsed local labour markets (Coles 1991, Jones 1993a). Class background and locality, Roberts argues, largely determine the type of school, the training scheme, or course of further education young people will attend and the labour market opportunities that they will be afforded. As well as class and locality, he recognized that sex and ethnicity further subdivided the three broad trajectories he described in terms of the types of jobs and training places which were attained. So, for instance, young women are described as destined to take up traditional clerical and caring female jobs, while young men are destined for manual trades or management.

Apart from one separate fringe project, the ESRC initiative, lamentably, did not include a systematic examination of the ways in which young people from different ethnic minorities experience the main transition processes of youth (Connolly et al. 1992). Yet a number of studies have pointed out that young people from such backgrounds have profoundly different experiences of education, training and the labour market to their white contemporaries (Bhat et al. 1988, Clough & Drew 1985, Skellington et al. 1992, Troyna & Smith 1983). Both Martin Mac an Ghaill and Heidi Safia Mirza, in studies of "black" groups of young people, outline the ways in which these experience schooling through forms of institutional racism (Mac an Ghaill 1988, Mirza 1992), and a number of studies have pointed to the under-performance of Afro-Caribbean boys, particularly, in terms of qualifications. Wrench has argued that they are also subject to "protective channelling" by the Careers Service which fails to confront the racial prejudice of employers, and a number of studies have further argued that young people from ethnic minorities are more likely to be placed on training schemes with the least chance of employment at the end (Solomos 1988, Verma & Darby 1987, Cross et al. 1990). In Mirza's study, young black women were described as unsubdued by their experience and highly ambitious in class terms, although this meant aspirations to gendered, and often poorly paid, careers in the caring professions (Mirza 1992). As Sillitoe & Meltzer demonstrate, young people from ethnic minorities are, therefore, most likely to experience the third of Roberts' three trajectories, though there is some indication that, perhaps understandably, they interpret this as confirming their beliefs about institutional racism in education, training and the labour market (Sillitoe & Meltzer 1985, Ullah 1985).

The qualitative (ethnographic) studies undertaken as part of the ESRC initiative describe the ways in which each of the main transitions are experienced by young people. These studies were undertaken in order to give access to the day-to-day experiences of young people in further education, on training schemes and in employment. In one sense they bear testimony to the active involvement of young people in shaping their own identities and, as such, it might be argued they do not present a picture of them as "cultural dopes" passively being propelled along pre-ordained "trajectories" (Bates & Riseborough 1993). The ethnographic studies describe how young people undertake an "extended socialization process" as they take part in Youth Training, further education or sixth-form studies. Roberts, of course, regards this as merely describing the processes through which young people are further locked into the main trajectories. The ethnographies show that taking part in some forms of education and training is often accompanied by rituals of resistance, rebellion and improvisation (Bates & Riseborough 1993). Yet, despite such patterns of resistance, girls taking courses in such subjects as fashion and design, for example, are eventually "snipped" down to size to suit the routine jobs they will be most likely to achieve in cutting out and making up other people's designs. Boys on catering courses, for instance, may laugh and joke about a boring, irrelevant and overly academic curriculum, but in the end they gain crucial "economic socialization" through either the part-time work experience they obtain for themselves or through work placements arranged by their college. Many of the girls training as care assistants are described as initially aiming for other, and more prestigious, gender-typified jobs, "working with children". But they are described as becoming locked into future careers in "care" occupations over time, through a reconstruction of their personal biographies and through adapting to the occupational culture of working with the elderly. Girls staying on into the sixth form of a private school are described as "gaining the edge" in terms of polish and poise as well as academic qualifications, as they move towards higher education and professional and managerial careers. Those being supported by public funding under the assisted places scheme, similarly integrate the values, behaviour and aspirations of their schoolmates in private schools. For Roberts, all these studies bear testimony to the fact that, while the everyday experiences of young people do allow some scope for decision making and agency, ultimately the career paths they follow illustrate the ways in which their lives are determined by the circumstances in which they find themselves.

Three further dimensions of disadvantage

As well as the four dimensions of difference listed on page 12 which have been argued to influence youth transitions, this book will document the ways in which three other structures of disadvantage are of fundamental importance. These have been largely ignored in the mainstream sociological literature describing the transition processes. The three are concerned with the impact of:
- being brought up in care
- having a disability, being in chronic ill health or defined as having "special needs"
- having been involved in crime and the criminal justice system.

While these three dimensions will not be of vital importance to all young people, they may have serious effects on others. All three were ignored by the ESRC study of *Careers and identities*. Yet each can be shown to be of critical importance in influencing youth transitions. As we will see in Chapter 6, young people who are brought up away from their biological families in local authority care suffer major disadvantages in education and later employment. Yet, as the chapter will also document, young people brought up in care are also much more likely to be required to live "independently" at a much earlier age than those brought up in their own families, and in this sense, despite their disadvantage in attempting the school-to-work transition, they are forced to attempt accelerated housing careers, compared to most of their contemporaries. Recent studies suggest that, at least in part as a result of this, they are highly likely to experience homelessness and are much more likely to be convicted of criminal offences and experience imprisonment (Anderson et al. 1993, Biehal et al. 1992, Garnett 1992).

The survey of the homeless undertaken for the Department of Environment, together with descriptions of the characteristics of the prison population, indicate just how debilitating poor health, care and imprisonment can be upon the main youth transitions (Anderson et al. 1993, Bines 1993). Research on both homelessness and imprisonment indicates a startling over-representation of young people who had been "in care". While those in care represent a tiny proportion of young people in each age group, a survey of homelessness conducted for the Department of the Environment found that one in four of those "sleeping rough" had spent some time in a children's home, and one in ten had lived in a foster home (Anderson et al. 1993). Furthermore, a survey of the prison population indicates that care leavers are vastly over-represented among those in prison, with 38% of prisoners having been in local authority care at some stage (Walmsley et al. 1992). The homelessness study further found that well over half of the young homeless had experienced either care, prison or time in a remand centre. Among the 16- and 17-year-old homeless, 54% of those in hostels for the homeless, 86% of those in day centres for the homeless, and 75% of those contacted through "soup runs" had either stayed with foster parents or been in at least one institution of care or custody (Anderson et al. 1993).

The impact of ill health can also be shown to be a major factor in the distribution of social and economic disadvantage and in "determining" failed or fractured transitions. If young people have no serious health problems then their health is unlikely to affect them in making the three main transitions. Where young persons have a physical or mental disability, however, as we will see in Chapter 7, this is likely to affect their opportunities in education and the type of training or employment they are likely to achieve. The Labour Force Surveys (LFSs) help to give some information about the fortunes of some vulnerable groups. The 1992 Labour Force Survey indicates that 14,000 16-year-olds and 21,000 17-year-olds (3 per cent of both the cohorts taken together) were said to be neither in full-time education, nor unemployed or "economically active". Of these, 13,000 were reported to be sick, injured or disabled or being looked after at home by their families (Sly 1993). As we will see in Chapter 7, disability is likely to have a major impact upon post-16 careers, influencing the type of activities to which young people will be directed and, where employed, their earning capacity. Disability also affects a young person's chances of leaving home and living independently. Disability thus influences all three of the main youth transitions. This means that young people with disabilities are most likely to experience "extended transitions" that often do not lead from school to work, but from school back to incarceration in the parental home. It is, therefore, a major determinant of both their "careers" and their future welfare.

The relationship between unemployment, crime and imprisonment is both complex and politically contentious (Coles & Fowles 1991, Crow 1989, Field 1990). Yet we know that young people in prison are more likely to have truanted from school and have achieved few (if any) qualifications (Farrington 1990). The status sequence from school to custody is therefore a most important one to examine and one which is followed by a significant minority of young people. The peak ages for offending are between the ages of 15 and 19 and by the age of 30 one in three young men has been convicted of a standard list of offences (Home Office Research and Statistics Dept. 1989). Yet the ESRC 16–19 Initiative study ignored this dimension of transition completely. When young people are convicted of a criminal offence, this may seriously affect their future employment career. Young people who are convicted of a serious offence or repeatedly offend are more likely to receive a custodial sentence and this, in turn, is likely seriously to disadvantage or exclude them from future participation in many segments of the labour market. As we will see in Chapter 8, where local legitimate opportunity structures are limited, and where unemployment levels are high, alternative and illegal opportunity structures are most likely to develop.

The importance of focusing on the concept of career

We now turn to the importance of retaining the concept of career as central to the development of a social policy of youth. While Roberts argues that the ESRC ethnographic studies describe the micro-social processes involved in youth "trajectories", they also have some resonance with the sociological concept of "career". In the 1960s Howard Becker, in developing the concept and applying it to the study of "deviance", argued that within the development of "deviant careers", there was a complex interaction between what people did (their activity), what people thought about what they were doing (their beliefs and justifications) and what they further learnt and practised as the activities and beliefs of the group (their social interactions) (Becker 1963). The Dartington Social Research Unit has further developed the concept in its examination of the impact of Youth Treatment Centres on the "careers" of young people after they leave such institutions (Bullock et al. 1994b). Authors from the unit have argued for the importance of understanding both the social and psychological processes set in train by each status, together with the impact of the decisions made by young people (and their families) and the support and control agencies in determining that status. They argue, with particular reference to highly disturbed young people, that "decisions made at successive moments of a career influences what happens subsequently". We will examine this in relationship to "criminal careers" in more detail in Chapter 8. But what is important to recognize here is the complexity of decision making involving young people, their parents, and other agencies responsible for their welfare. For many young people, it is these negotiated or imposed decisions which determine each discrete stage in a status sequence, and which set in train a whole range of social and psychological processes associated with the incumbency of each status position. This involves, what Becker called, a series of "activities", "beliefs and justifications" and "interactions", which further help to determine the likelihood of moving to each future status position within a "career" development. It is because of this that Becker wished to retain the importance of treating "career" as a process, rather than seeing activity as a socially "determined" behavioural outcome.

In the context of this understanding of the concept of "career", and the leverage this can give us on understanding the progression from one status to another, the ethnographic studies undertaken as part of the ESRC project do much more than add weight and "meaning" to three main "trajectories". For, in concentrating on "social and psychological processes", they illustrate the important interplay between all sides of the "career equation"; the structuration and changing shape of opportunity structures and the agency of all those involved in making choices about young people's careers. In some circumstances it is young people themselves who choose particular career options to follow, and some of them can, and do, choose to give them up. In other circumstances, adults make decisions by acting as "gatekeepers" of welfare institutions, steering young people towards new statuses which are deemed appropriate. In seeking to retrieve the concept of "career" from an over-deterministic concept of "trajectory", this book seeks to focus attention not only upon the "choices" young people may or may not have, but on the responsibilities a variety of youth professionals also have, in determining young people's welfare. Using the concept of "career" also has the benefit of focusing attention on the possibilities for change rather than the inevitability of pessimistic outcomes. But this point should be accompanied by a word of caution. In arguing for the importance of the concept of career, it is not the intention to supplant the profound influence of social background in shaping the opportunity structures of the young with some innocent or voluntaristic notion of free choice and individual agency. Rather, it is to insist that we must give due regard to both sides of the equation.

Ultimately, whichever status young persons may attain, and whatever social group they may join at each stage of the post-16 transition, they may ultimately have a "choice" as to whether to stay or leave. For those in secure accommodation even that choice is limited. Where young persons are students studying a particular course, they may have only one simple choice, to stay or to leave. Yet even this is a real choice of real consequence. A 1993 Audit Commission report on young people in full-time post-16 education indicated that between 30% and 40% of young people either drop out of their course or do not succeed in attaining the qualification (Audit Commission–OFSTED 1993). In the next chapter we will examine the background to the growth of post-16 education which Roberts dismisses as a mere mirage of changed opportunities. It seems disingenuous to recognize the potential impact of each and every status position to set in motion distinct patterns of extended socialization, to recognize that these have grown in both number, size and complexity in the late 1980s and 1990s, and yet to regard such major structural changes as no more than a cosmetic rearrangement within three main "trajectories". This book seeks to reassert the importance of the concept of career as against an overly deterministic concept of trajectory. This is not, of course, to deny that the changing shape of the labour market has an impact upon the occupational careers young people will eventually achieve. Changes in education and training do not create extra or different jobs. But in responding to the opportunities that education, training and the labour market offer them, young people do choose between different career options. Of course they are influenced by those around them, especially parents and friends (Killeen et al. 1992). But they can also be influenced by more formal agencies of careers education and guidance (Coles 1993). While it may be understandable that sociologists, wishing to explain broad patterns of social reproduction, resort to an over-simplistic modelling of youth transitions through determinist concepts such as trajectory, it is important that the social policy of youth conceptualizes the transitions in ways which can address the possibility of change. It is, after all, part of the *raison d'être* of social policy to seek out aspects of policy intervention whereby change (and improvement) can be realized. It is for all these reasons that we must focus attention on the concept of career.

The concept of career has a long history within sociological literature and is of particular importance to our understanding of youth in several different ways. First, as we have seen, it helps us understand the transitions of youth as a series of status sequences which are both chosen by young people, but only from within a set of alternatives which are structurally determined. The concept of youth careers, thus, allows us to examine the interplay between structuration and agency; the relationship between institutional and structural development and young people as active agents who respond to structural changes rather than being simply driven along by them. Secondly, the concept allows us to examine how choices made at one point in the transition are capable of both opening up and closing down the possibility of attaining future career moves. As we have seen, this is most obvious in the case of education, training and labour market careers, where decisions at the age of 16 about education and training determine which segments of the labour market young people may be qualified to join at some future point. But this is not a return to the concept of trajectory, since the determination is based upon a choice made by young people at a previous point in the status sequence.

Thirdly, the concept of career allows for a clearer recognition that youth transitions are multidimensional. Much of the work on youth trajectories has been confined to an examination of the links between education, training and occupation. Yet, as we have seen, there was a recognition of the ways in which locality trapped some young people within an area which offered few job opportunities. In this sense education is not merely a potential vehicle of occupational and social mobility but of geographical mobility too. As MacDonald has argued, "getting on" (through education) is often undertaken as a means of "getting out" (of the restricted options available in local labour markets) (MacDonald 1988). Higher education has been recognized as offering not merely the chance of education after the age of 18, and subsequently a chance to seek a job in an (inter)national graduate labour market, but also as a means through which young people embark upon a "housing career" – moving away from their family of origin by being offered accommodation at their place of learning (Jones 1987). The foyers system, as developed in France, similarly offers young people there the chance to escape from their locality to undertake work or training by offering them, at the same time, accommodation away from home (Heddy 1991). A similar system is being developed in Britain (Baldwin 1994, Chatrik 1994a, Quilgars & Anderson 1993). Despite some major reservations about the implementation of this scheme in Britain, in theory at least, foyers present a more imaginative approach to policy intervention which recognizes the interrelationship between occupation and training needs and the associated need for appropriate housing provision. In this sense, it offers an opportunity to break through the no home, no job cycle.

Fourthly, it should be recognized that the sociological concept of career does not imply that the status sequences it identifies brings with it advancement or progress. It may, indeed, bring a diminution of welfare. For just as Becker, in the 1960s, was able to talk of the "moral career" of drug users as they became more and more firmly involved in a drug culture, an examination of housing career might also map routes into street homelessness (Hutson & Liddiard 1991, Jones 1993b), while other studies of "deviant career" describe routes into persistent crime, including lengthy periods in various forms of custody (Little 1990, Bullock et al. 1994a). Similarly, occupational careers include not only those which involve increases in skill, levels of responsibility and pay, but some "careers" may lead from training to bouts of unemployment, to casual work, and back to unemployment, further training, and perhaps finally to longer-term joblessness. It is the task of a social policy for youth, not only to describe the depressingly determined trajectories, but to devise policies which can either help prevent these worst scenarios from happening or offer routes back from the failed and fractured transitions.

Finally, as we map the various interrelated elements of young careers, what becomes clear is that the consequences of each successive stage in a status sequence is a change in the welfare afforded to, or achieved by, the young person concerned. In examining the "careers" of young people who left Youth Treatment Centres, for instance, the Dartington Social Research Unit examined the multifaceted aspects of their future lives including their home circumstances, their employment, their physical and psychological health, their dependency on state institutions, as well as patterns of future offending (Bullock et al. 1994a). In this sense, the examination of the interlocking nature of youth transitions also helps to map an overall "welfare career", where welfare implies a whole complex of rights, needs, interests, benefits and material circumstances. This aggregated "welfare career" for young people can also be seen as being related to the attainment (or denial) of aspects of citizenship which will be examined in more detail in Chapters 4 and 5.

The transitions of youth we have described can, therefore, be regarded as being akin to a rather vicious version of the board game "snakes and ladders". The three main transitions are the ladders through which young people gradually move towards adult statuses. Those young people who come from stable, secure and advantaged home backgrounds may have extended transitions through education before entering the labour market and attempting permanent housing and partner transitions and, as we shall see in the next two chapters, the ladders available to them have been restructured and rearranged over the past two decades. Those disadvantaged by social class background; those brought up in localities in which local labour markets offer few opportunities for employment; those brought up in care; those who suffer problems with their health or have special needs; those who become involved in the criminal justice system; all these groups are prone to sliding down the "snakes" in the transition game and to suffer serious set-backs in their attempts to move towards adult status and relative independency and autonomy. For if, as we shall see in the next two chapters, youth has been restructured in the last quarter of a century, it is the vulnerable who have suffered the most in coping with the transitions associated with these changes.

The cost of youth policy failures

It is not within the scope of this text to calculate the exact cost of policy failures, but it is perhaps important to point to some indicators of failure which could be used, and to highlight some of the huge savings which could be made, if policies were more effectively targeted at better managing the transitions of youth. When young people leave 11 years of compulsory education without any formal qualifications, it is not just they who have "failed", it is the education policies which have cost more than £20 billion of public expenditure each year. Where young people fail to achieve any qualifications at the age of 16 and do so having been brought up in the care of public authorities, and when they later become homeless or resort to crime, this indicates that the state has acted like the worst parents in the country and at a huge expense to social service budgets (*Independent* 13 November 1993). When young people leave special education only to find themselves directed to a lifetime in day centres and Adult Training Centres rather than forms of protected and supported employment schemes, this too is to add billions of pounds to social service budgets. When a hundred thousand young people leave school and do not secure employment and are not offered places on schemes of Youth Training, they may not be able to claim Income Support, but they are highly likely to be set on a career which will involve long-term unemployment (Convery & Taylor 1993). Over a million people in Britain have been unemployed for a year or more, with an estimated cost to the Exchequer of between £9,000 and £10,000 each. The estimated cost of unemployment in 1992–3 was a staggering £21.5 billion, taking into account benefit payments and lost income from tax and national insurance (Taylor 1993). Furthermore, this does not take into account further associated costs of the health care of the unemployed or the "crime costs" should they resort to illegal means of making a living. One calculation of the cost of youth crime put it as £7 billion per year (*Independent* 22 September 1994). Another calculation suggests that for each 1 per cent rise in unemployment there is a correlated rise in the imprisonment of young offenders and an extra bill for £1 million to be met by the Home Office (Coles & Fowles 1991). When young people drift into crime, this results in costs to those against whom the crime is committed, to others thought to be vulnerable to crime (because of increased insurance costs), and eventually to the tax payer, through the cost of court proceedings and (if necessary) custody. The estimated average weekly cost of keeping one young person in secure accommodation for one week is £1,680 (House of Commons 1993), and as high as £2,700 in some Youth Treatment Centres (*Independent* 7 May 1994). To keep hundreds more in such accommodation for up to two years, as suggested by the Home Secretary in 1993, will add further billions of pounds to public expenditure. Yet, unqualified school-leavers, unemployment, crime and imprisonment are not the only costs to be considered. For example, suicides among young men have nearly doubled in the past two decades (Woodroffe et al. 1993). The costs of adequately addressing the youth policy areas covered in this book are considerable. But the costs of not doing so are also huge. It will be argued throughout this book, that we can no longer afford to fail young people with social policies we design for their welfare. It is time for us to take our responsibilities seriously.

Part One

Towards a framework
for youth policy

Chapter Two

The re-structuration of youth: the school-to-work transition

Chapter 1 outlined a conceptualization of youth based on a series of "transitions" from childhood to adulthood. These transitions, of course, have changed in pattern over time in terms of the age at which young people attempt to make them and the difficulties they may encounter. The next two chapters describe a number of ways in which social and economic structures which frame youth transitions have been fundamentally transformed in the last quarter of the twentieth century. For the majority of young people in the United Kingdom, the time at which they now leave full-time education, their economic dependency on their parents, and their first moves away from the parental home have all been subject to the influence of economic and social changes which have occurred in the last two decades. These structural shifts have both restructured the nature and meaning of "youth" and significantly reshaped the welfare environment in which young people grow up. The next two chapters focus on the "re-structuration" of youth in the sense that we will examine *both* the social and economic institutions which frame young people's lives, *and* the changing patterns of choices which young people and their families make in responding to the changing world around them. The chapters focus upon the three main transitions outlined in Chapter 1: the school-to-work transition; the relationship between young people and families; and the ways in which both these affect "housing careers" as young people move away from the parental home.

This chapter will draw upon a number of large-scale social surveys which describe the conditions under which young people grow up in the United Kingdom. These include "cross-sectional" snap shots of particular institutions (such as the labour market, family or education). Other surveys attempt to be longitudinal and follow representative samples of young people as they move through various stages in their life cycle. One of these latter surveys is the National Child Development Study (NCDS) which traces the fortunes of all babies born during a single week in 1958 and has collected data about their circumstances at the ages of 7, 11, 16, 23 and 33. The cohort reached their late teens in the latter half of the 1970s. Most young people then seemed to manage youth transitions with relative ease and at an early age (Kiernan 1992). Kiernan reports that by 1976, when the cohort had reached the age of 18, more than two-thirds of them had left school and got a job. Indeed, most left school at the minimum school-leaving age of 16 and nine out of ten had secured employment within six months of leaving. It is now widely recognized that leaving school and earning a wage carried symbolic importance for both young people and their parents. Once young people become wage earners, their parents seem to regard them as "grown-up" and adult and, as a result, give them more responsibilities and freedoms (Coffield et al. 1986, Coles 1986, Willis 1984). For those leaving school in the mid-1970s, earning a wage also allowed many of them to marry and move away from the parental home by their early 20s. Kiernan reports that, by the age of 21, half the NCDS sample had left home and more than a third of young women were married (Kiernan 1992).

Since the 1970s, however, this picture has changed dramatically. Much of this has been prompted by the growth of youth unemployment and changes in the youth labour market. The changing patterns of employment have also resulted in new and different patterns of leaving home and family formation (Jones 1987, Jones & Wallace 1992, Wallace 1987). Compared to youth transitions in the 1970s, by the mid-1990s all three youth transitions have become more complex, take longer periods of time, and prove much more difficult to accomplish successfully. In this sense, many young people in the 1990s experience either "extended" or "fractured" transitions. Extended transitions refer to the fact that the attainment of employment, leaving home and setting up new households in the 1990s is much more likely to take place at a later age than in previous decades. Extended transitions from school to work also mean that young people are economically dependent upon their families for longer periods of time, and for some this places great strain on family relationships. As we will see in the next chapter, this is exacerbated by changes in family structures and family relationships. Fractured transitions refer to situations in which young people move from one status position, without managing to attain a secure, stable or positive outcome in another. So, for instance, young people may leave education but not obtain a job; they may leave their families without entering into other permanent households; they may leave home without attaining another form of permanent housing. At their worst, fractured transitions result in long-term and chronic unemployment, dislocation and estrangement from families, and homelessness (Williamson 1993).

As youth transitions have changed in the last two decades, different groups of young people have been affected in different ways. In the last chapter, it was pointed out that sociologists have long argued that patterns of youth transition differ significantly according to social class background, gender, ethnic group, region and locality (Banks et al. 1992, Jones & Wallace 1992). We further signalled that other forms of disadvantage could accrue from having a special educational need, a physical or mental disability, being brought up in the care of local authorities or involved in the criminal justice system. These will be examined in Chapters 6–8. As we describe structural changes in the labour market and education and training systems in this chapter, it should be recognized that these have a differential effect on different groups. Some may be argued to have benefited from institutional reforms and widening opportunities (such as the expansion of post-16 education). Other young people have experienced structural change as resulting in their progressive marginalization and social exclusion from the opportunity structures of mainstream society. As such, some of the changes we describe can be regarded as leading to the manufacture of more acute inequalities of opportunity (Williamson 1993).

The growth of youth unemployment and developments in (un)employment policy

Of all the changes which have affected the lives of young people in the latter stages of the twentieth century, it is the return of mass unemployment in the 1980s which can be argued to have had the most far-reaching consequences. Even its definition has become politically contentious, with over thirty changes in the ways in which the official count has been undertaken since the election of the first government of Mrs Thatcher in 1979 (Metcalf 1992). Since 1982, the official unemployment count for the United Kingdom has been based upon the numbers of people out of work *and* in receipt of benefit, rather than out of work and actively seeking it, even though this latter definition is more commonly accepted internationally. The UK Labour Force Survey (LFS), however, continues to collect unemployment data according to the internationally accepted definition. Pissarides & Wadsworth have calculated that, while in 1979 the Labour Force Survey estimates of the rates of unemployment and the claimant count were very similar, by 1989 the official unemployment rate accounted for only 68 per cent of the unemployed as defined by internationally recognized criteria (Pissarides & Wadsworth 1992). Despite the official count of unemployment persistently approaching 3 million or more since the early 1980s, the official figures significantly underestimate the extent of unemployment (McLaughlin 1994).

According to the international definition of unemployment, the rate among those under 25 in Great Britain was as low as 2.4% in 1960, 5.9% in 1970, had risen to 12.2% by 1979, but reached 21.4% by 1981 (Ashton 1986). Young people have traditionally been the most vulnerable to general trends in unemployment and this certainly proved to be the case in the 1970s (Makeham 1980). Roberts, for instance, estimated that between 1972 and 1977, whereas general unemployment rose by 45%, unemployment among 16–17-year-olds increased by 120% (Roberts 1984). Estimates based on the 1993 Labour Force Survey suggest that, while the general unemployment rate was 10.2%, unemployment among 16–24-year-olds stood at 17.5% (Sly 1993). Yet even this apparently simple statement about the extent of unemployment among 16–24-year-olds underestimates the potential problem. For while young people may indeed be more vulnerable to unemployment, many more of this age group – more than in previous decades – are sheltering within the education and training systems and, therefore, have still to start seeking work.

Young people growing up in the 1980s and 1990s have experienced a world in which mass unemployment has constantly been on the agenda. Their response suggests that they are unwilling merely to be passive victims of structures beyond their control. Knowing that there are fewer jobs for 16-year-olds, and that qualifications beyond those gained at 16 may give them a better chance of a more secure and desirable job, many more now stay within education for longer (Department for Education 1993). The indirect effect of mass unemployment, therefore, has been to displace young people into training and education. As we will see, this displacement has taken different forms at different periods of time. Ashton and others have argued that, until 1979, youth unemployment was largely confined to un-qualified school-leavers (Ashton 1986, Casson 1979, Roberts 1984). During the 1979–85 recession, as unemployment among 16–25-year-olds rose to a quarter of all school-leavers, a much wider group was affected. In the 1980s, this group became displaced into various forms of Youth Training. In the late 1980s and 1990s, however, Youth Training declined in popularity to be replaced by an increasing tendency for young people to stay in education beyond minimum school-leaving age. Labour market trends and forecasts indicate that several shifts in the nature of work have now taken a strong hold, and that these, taken together, imply that young people will enter the labour market at a later stage in their lives, will be expected to be much better educated and trained, and can expect to experience both unemployment, retraining and a change of career at several points in their working lives (Ashton et al. 1990, Beck 1992). Until recently, policy makers have resisted any assumption that we can return to "full employment" (for exceptions see Commission on Social Justice 1994, Field 1993). It is little wonder, therefore, that faced with the fear of unemployment – through the career choices they make at the ages of 16 and 18 – young people have contributed to the changing pattern of the school-to-work transition, and changed tack according to what they see as their most secure route to a stable and prosperous economic future.

Since 1979, the policy response to unemployment under successive Conservative governments has been limited by an overriding commitment to bring down inflation and curb public expenditure. There has been an acceptance that it is only from private enterprise that any sustainable upturn in labour demand will come. Repeatedly, government White Papers have argued that the duty of the government was to "set a climate" for economic growth and recovery rather than embark upon direct action through public expenditure to create jobs (Department of Employment 1988). So, for instance, the White Paper *Employment for the 1990s* was couched in terms of breaking down "barriers to employment". By this was meant: reforming "industrial relations" (reducing too-high pay demands); improving training (remedying the skill-mismatch between labour supply and demand); and reducing work disincentives (remedying the belief that a person was better off on benefit than in work). More specific policy initiatives have been directed to four main areas of concern: interest rate and inflation policies to stimulate private industrial investment; a reduction in the power of the unions in wage bargaining so as, supposedly, to price workers into jobs; some limited intervention and support to the regions most affected by unemployment, to encourage inward investment and economic development; and support for education and training programmes. This latter policy has been deemed necessary so as to keep the unemployed and those at school and college motivated to train and seek work and to keep them "in circulation" (by being effectively warehoused in education or on training schemes).

Policies directed at *youth* unemployment can be argued to have taken place along four broad fronts. The first and most visible form of intervention was the development and expansion of a number of different training schemes for 16- and 17-year-olds during the growth of unemployment in the 1970s and 1980s (Gleeson 1989, Raffe 1988, Rees & Atkinson 1982, Roberts 1984, Wallace & Cross 1990). At the height of recession in the mid-1980s, the Youth Training Scheme (YTS) recruited more than a quarter (28%) of all 16-year-olds (Jones et al. 1988). The proportion of young people in each age group prepared to take part in Youth Training in its various guises has, however, fluctuated markedly since then, and by 1991 the Youth Cohort Study of England and Wales (YCS) reported that only 14% of 16–17-year-olds were taking part in Youth Training (Courtnay & McAleese 1993b). A second area of policy intervention concerned the regulation of the youth labour market itself and a drive towards encouraging this to be "more flexible". This, it was argued, would allow young people to price themselves into work. This formed a main defence against attempts made under the Social Chapter of the Maastricht Treaty to introduce minimum wages and more controlled conditions of employment (Employment Department 1992). As we will see, there is some evidence this increased "flexibility" in the youth labour market has been achieved. But any real growth of labour market opportunities for young people can be argued to take the form either of part-time work for young people still in full-time education, or, for those who obtain full-time employment, to have been achieved only at the cost of reducing average youth wages and weakening young people's conditions of employment.

The reform of education, and in particular the expansion of post-16 educational opportunities, constitutes a third front of policy development. This has included a number of major changes introduced under the 1988 Education Reform Act. As well as these, a number of initiatives in vocational education were introduced both before and after the 1988 Act. Furthermore, changes in the curricula and assessment of 16-plus qualification and the subsequent expansion of post-16 participation rates have also had a major influence on the school-to-work transition (Gray et al. 1993). Fourthly, as more young people were displaced from the labour market into education and training, the government sought to intensify these trends by changing the social security system. Following the Fowler reviews of social security in the mid-1980s, young people's entitlement to social security benefits and other forms of welfare support has been considerably reduced (Craig 1991, Harris 1989). These modifications of social security arrangements constitute a fourth important area of policy change. Taken together, these four policy developments have had a very far-reaching impact upon the structures of opportunity in which young people develop their "careers". Each of these four policy fronts will be examined and assessed in turn.

The growth and expansion of Youth Training

As the National Child Development Study testifies, until the mid-1970s, most young people in Britain left school at the minimum school-leaving age and went into a full-time job (Kiernan 1992). The economic recession during the latter half of the 1970s and the early 1980s all but destroyed this simple, predominant, and one-step transition from school to work. Roberts, among others, has commented upon the suddenness of the change. "In 1974 sixty one per cent of Britain's 16 year olds were employed. In 1984 only 18% had jobs.

Hence the talk of the 'vanishing youth labour market' " (Coles 1988: 23). By the mid-1990s, only one in eight 16-year-olds had a full-time job (Courtnay & McAleese 1993b). Despite the ebbs and flows of further economic recessions and recovery, the youth labour market as it existed in the early 1970s has not re-emerged.

In the 1970s and 1980s, what replaced the simple transition from school to work at the age of 16 was the growth of both youth unemployment and "extended transitions" made via Youth Training Schemes, in part designed to ameliorate the worst effects of unemployment. Initially, at the beginning of the 1970s, "special measures" were introduced which were largely composed of either 12-week courses of work experience, or financial inducements to employers to employ 16-year-olds (Rees & Atkinson 1982). As youth unemployment continued to grow, these schemes became "rationalized" under the proposals of the Holland Report into a six-month long Youth Opportunities Programme (YOP) introduced in 1978 under a Labour government (Manpower Services Commission 1977). The Holland Report envisaged that YOP would have to cater for up to half a million young people and the aim of YOP was to offer training and work experience and to stagger the entry of school-leavers to the labour market over the six-month period following summer school-leaving. Yet, in the late 1970s, youth unemployment continued to grow at an alarming rate and young people resisted recruitment on to YOP, regarding it as poorly paid "slave labour" and doing little to help them secure employment (Rees & Atkinson 1982, Roberts 1984). Government response to resistance to YOP was a longer training scheme which claimed to offer a higher quality of training. Following the 1981 White Paper *A new training initiative*, YOP was replaced by a twelve-month Youth Training Scheme (YTS) in 1983 (Manpower Services Commission 1981). This was extended to a two-year programme YTS2 in 1985. Youth Training had thus been increased in length more than eightfold in five years (Coles & MacDonald 1990). Furthermore, while the early courses of work experience accounted for only a small minority of, largely unqualified, school-leavers, by the mid-1980s YTS catered for more than a quarter of the age group and thus included young people with a variety of different levels of school qualification (Ashton 1986). A further revision of Youth Training initiatives took place in 1991 with the introduction of Youth Training (YT). This was intended to be more focused towards the attainment of National Vocational Qualifications (NVQs) (Ainley 1991). By the mid-1990s many of these programmes were being run under brand names, in part at least, to distance them from the poor reputation previous schemes had had with young people and their parents.

Much has been written about the growth of Youth Training and much of the detail need not concern us here (Finn 1987, Gleeson 1983, 1989, Hollands 1990, Lee et al. 1990, Raffe 1988). But some features of its expansion are important to note. First, the training allowances paid to young people have always been considerably less than wage rates paid to young workers by employers. In the late 1970s and early 1980s under YOP, trainee allowances were regularly up-rated, but stood at only £23.50 per week in 1981 (Rees & Atkinson 1982). Throughout the 1980s, despite rises in wage levels, youth trainee allowances have remained very low relative to jobs outside of YTS. Under Youth Training, introduced in 1991, employers were encouraged to give trainees employment status and to top up their training allowances. Yet the Youth Cohort Study of England and Wales estimated that in 1991 young men on YT had an average take-home pay of £39.00 and young women £37.35, compared with wage rates of young workers employed outside YT where young men of the same age had an average take-home pay of £79.70 and young women a slightly higher average of £81.70 (Courtnay & McAleese 1993b). One estimate suggests that, had the Youth Training allowance been upgraded in line with other wage rates, by the mid-1990s it would have been in excess of £70 per week (Unemployment Unit–Youthaid, March 1994). Since the early days of YOP the most persistent criticism of schemes by young people is that they are "slave labour" (Hughes 1984, MacDonald 1988, White & Brockington 1983). By the end of the 1980s, they had a firmly established reputation among young people and their parents as something to be taken only if all else failed (Coles 1991, 1993). The Youth Cohort Studies confirm that, while young people are positive in the way in which they regard the work, training and social contacts which they made through their training scheme, YT participants were three times more likely to complain about low pay than their contemporaries in employment outside YT. Four out of ten respondents in full-time work, and over a quarter of those unemployed, had turned down a YT place because the pay was considered to be too low (Courtnay & McAleese 1993b).

Secondly, while YOP, YTS and YT were initially marketed as a single government scheme, there have always been clear differences between schemes offered by different sponsors, employers and managers. Young people have recognized this and acted accordingly. David Raffe has suggested that a clear stratification system existed even in the mid-1980s (Raffe 1986). At the top end, the most prestigious and sought-after schemes (in the "sponsorship" sector) were run by employers. These proved the most likely to lead to employment when the scheme came to an end. At the other end of the spectrum were schemes in the "detached" sector – schemes often run by local authorities or charities and based in workshops or training centres. These latter schemes often catered for the least qualified or most vulnerable and, no matter how good the training provided, proved to be the least successful in placing trainees in permanent employment at the end. In between were other schemes which served to put young people in touch with "real" employers during work placements or trained them in specific skills which were in demand in the local labour market. What is increasingly clear is that, despite all the revisions and changes made to Youth Training since the mid-1980s, these divisions still exist in the mid-1990s. Some training hostels (which offer both accommodation for the homeless and training) continue to replicate the training offered in the "detached" sector of the 1980s, whereas major employers are attempting to emphasize their "sponsorship role" by distancing themselves from the very name Youth Training and using brand names of their own (Baldwin 1994). These latter schemes now make it difficult for some young workers to know whether they are taking part in YT at all (Courtnay & McAleese 1993b).

Thirdly, in the 1990s, youth trainees are clustered in a limited number of occupational areas. These closely resemble the youth labour market which, as we will see, is also deeply "segmented" by occupational area and gender. Ashton, among others, has commented on the way in which labour markets often have clearly defined segments which, because of similarities of training and experience, allow mobility between jobs but only limited possibilities of job mobility between segments (Ashton 1986, Ashton et al. 1990). The Youth Cohort Studies (YCS) indicate that the occupational areas in which youth trainees find training places in the 1990s very closely match the segments in which young people found work outside YT.

Furthermore, both the jobs and training places they obtained indicate that opportunities were clearly stratified by gender. In the YCS study of young people reaching the age of 16 in 1991, more than four-fifths of young women on YT were being trained in clerical, cleaning, catering or selling jobs, while three-quarters of their contemporaries in jobs outside YT were in the same occupational categories. While young men had a wider mix of jobs and training places, just over half of 16-year-olds in work or training clustered in three segments: construction, mining and manufacturing. Slightly more (55%) of those on Youth Training were to be found in these sectors compared with those in work outside YT (51%) (Courtnay & McAleese 1993b). What this means is that while Youth Training is often marketed as a bridge to work, it is only a bridge to certain types of gender-typified jobs. Many of these are in a very limited range of occupations and, as we will see, many traditional youth jobs simply disappeared as full-time jobs in the 1980s.

Fourthly, a number of studies conducted in the 1980s indicated that the collapse of job opportunities, and the subsequent growth in both unemployment and Youth Training, did not take place evenly across the country. Perhaps one of the more startling findings by Ashton and his colleagues was that, in the early 1980s, a young man's chance of being unemployed in Sunderland (a high unemployment area in North-East England) was one in three, compared with one in thirty-three in the prosperous southern town of St Albans (Ashton et al. 1988). This local labour market effect confounded even the other major predictors of labour market success or failure, such as social class background or qualifications gained at school. Armed with this knowledge, the ESRC series of studies of youth transitions in the late 1980s attempted to examine the impact of locality (Banks et al. 1992). These studies found that in the early 1980s, in the manufacturing areas of the North of England and the Midlands, unemployment grew much more rapidly than in the South and the proportion of young people leaving school to join Youth Training Schemes grew in response. In high unemployment areas, like Liverpool and Sheffield in the late 1980s, the collapse of the youth labour market displaced young school-leavers into training, with around half reported as joining YTS (Banks et al. 1992). Some youth trainees obtained employment at the end of their scheme but the majority merely delayed unemployment until the age of 18. In more prosperous towns like

Swindon in the South, the simple school-to-work transition at 16 still proved possible for nearly 30% of the age group in the late 1980s, while another 30% went on to YTS (Banks et al. 1992). The growth of Youth Training, particularly in the 1980s, thus extended the traditional transition from school to work for a substantial number of young people, but merely delayed unemployment for others.

A fifth important factor to note about Youth Training is that, by the 1990s, youth trainees had distinct educational and social background characteristics. The Youth Cohort Study of the sample of people reaching the age of 16 in 1991 reports that youth trainees are very unlikely to be well qualified, with only 3% of the group having four or more GCSEs above grade C. A quarter of those in YT reported they had no qualifications and a further 29% did not answer the question. Youth Training is also less popular among young women, partly perhaps because young women get better qualifications than young men do at the age of 16 and therefore have a choice as to whether to leave or stay on in post-16 education. But part of their reluctance to join YT may be the result of the traineeships only offering a very restricted range of gender-typified jobs with limited prospects. By the early 1990s, when youth traineeships were in short supply in many areas, those who left school for YT were more than twice as likely to be white rather than a member of an ethnic minority group (Courtnay & McAleese 1993b). Young people from Asian backgrounds were as likely as their white contemporaries to be unemployed. On the other hand, those identifying themselves as black or in an "other non-white" ethnic group were nearly twice as likely to be unoccupied; they were neither in education, nor in work or training. The Youth Cohort Studies also collect information on the social class background of their respondents, although such information is often difficult to collect or treat as reliable. The studies have also changed the classification systems they have used, so comparison between cohorts is difficult. However, what is clear is that those young people on YT in the 1990s were highly likely to have parents in semi- or unskilled occupational groups, and that their occupational class background continued to resemble most that of those who had also left school at 16 and obtained employment (Courtnay and McAleese 1993b). The extension of the school-to-work transition through Youth Training, therefore, is a feature of working-class, but not middle-class, life.

Changes in the structure of the youth labour market in the 1990s

The growth of Youth Training is not only linked to youth unemployment but also to the restructuring of the labour market more generally. Ashton and his colleagues have provided a detailed analysis of the complexity of these changes (Ashton et al. 1990). As they indicate, during the 1980s some types of youth employment and apprenticeships had become submerged under training schemes, as employers found it advantageous to use government-subsidized schemes rather than directly employ young people outside of Youth Training. Yet, during the 1970s and 1980s, some youth jobs simply disappeared, overtaken by shifts in manufacturing techniques and growing technology (Ashton et al. 1990, Roberts et al. 1987). Ashton and his colleagues have further calculated that apprenticeships reduced in number from nearly a quarter of a million places in the mid-1960s to only around 55,000 by the end of the 1980s. The proportion of young men in apprenticeships also fell during the same period, from just short of 6% to just over 2%, and the proportion of young women in formal apprenticeships had dwindled to only 1% (Ashton et al. 1989).

The Youth Cohort Study survey data also help to understand the pattern of movement into the youth labour market, the structure of the labour market itself and the ways in which early school-leavers are clustered in only particular occupational segments. At the time of the first survey in England and Wales, which studied those who reached minimum school-leaving age in 1984, the 16–17-year-olds who obtained jobs clustered in sectors or segments known as "KOS" (key occupational groups for statistical purposes). In 1984, nearly a third (31%) of boys, and just over a quarter of young women (25%) obtained a full-time job outside of YTS. Yet three-quarters of the young women who did so got jobs in a restricted cluster of occupations, which included clerical or secretarial work, catering, cleaning and personal services such as hair dressing or work in shops. The young men who found work outside of YTS obtained a wider range of occupations, although material processing accounted for four out of ten of them. As the study followed the 1984 cohort further into their careers, a greater proportion entered the labour market. By February 1987, 60% of young men and 57% of young women were in employment. Yet the types of jobs they had obtained clustered in similar sectors. Nearly four out of ten young men (38%) of those who had jobs obtained them in material processing, with the rest scattered widely through the range of industrial sectors. Nearly half (47%) of young women had clerical and secretarial jobs and a further 17% were involved in catering or cleaning. Obtaining jobs in "selling" was largely achieved by young women leaving school at minimum school-leaving age rather than being reserved for later leavers. At the beginning of the 1990s, the youth labour market had shrunk but had not otherwise changed very significantly. Among those who reached minimum school-leaving age in 1991, less than a quarter of young men (22%) obtained employment outside of YT, with jobs in manufacturing or construction and mining accounting for more than half (51%) of them. Only one in seven young women (14%) had a job outside YT, with this smaller group again being clustered in the same KOS categories as in the previous decade. Three-quarters (75%) of young women reported that they were employed in clerical or secretarial work, catering, cleaning and personal services or in selling. What appears to have happened in the late 1980s and 1990s is that, while the same broad occupational sectors predominated, fewer young people entered the full-time labour market, and even less are now joining programmes of Youth Training. The rerouting of the school-to-work transition through training only had a marginal effect on the type of jobs young people eventually obtained. For many it merely delayed the age at which they got them.

This segmentation of the youth labour market is also confirmed by data from Labour Force Surveys. Interestingly, the 1992 survey also reports on the economic activity of those who were also in full-time education, which allows us to examine the youth labour market in much broader terms (Sly 1993). Table 2.1 summarizes the main findings. One of the fastest-growing areas of employment in the late 1980s and early 1990s has been in part-time jobs. Until recently, little was known about the involvement of young people in part-time work, but the analysis of recent Labour Force Survey data allows us to examine both its extent and its significance. The 1992 Labour Force Survey confirms that relatively few 16- and 17-year-olds were in full-time employment. In the winter of 1992–3, of the 1.3 million 16- and 17-year-olds, only 312,000 were employed and not in full-time education. This indicates that less than a quarter of the two year groups were either in full-time work or undertaking YT. On the other hand, over 300,000 16–17-year-olds, nearly as many as were working full-time, were working while still in full-time education.

Table 2.1   16–17-year-olds in employment by industry and occupation.

	In full time education	Not in full time education
Numbers in '000s	305	312
Percentage of each group by industry		
Manufacturing/extraction	6	24
Construction	–	8
Distribution/hotels & catering	78	31
Other services	15	28
Percentage of each group by occupation		
Managerial/professional	2	5
Clerical/secretarial	5	14
Craft and related	–	24
Personal, protective	17	13
Selling	43	13
Plant/machine operatives	–	7
Other occupations	29	13

Source: Sly 1993, table 2.

As we have already seen, some forms of employment have been restructured with more and more part-time jobs replacing those previously offered to young full-time workers. Table 2.1 indicates that a considerable number of young people in full-time education are also involved in employment, particularly in distribution, hotel and catering, selling and providing a variety of other services. Some of this expansion of part-time employment has been taken up by students still in full-time post-16 education, some of whom can earn as much through part-time working as those on YT (Coles 1991). Most 16–17-year-olds engaged in both education and employment worked less than 10 hours per week (although 47% worked between 5 and 10 hours in each week). More than a quarter (28%) worked between 10 and 20 hours, while 5% worked over 20 hours per week while still being full-time students.

The law and protection of children and young people at work
Until recently, little was written about the paid work undertaken by children and young people still at school and college, but this is an

important part of the jigsaw which makes up the picture of young people's relationship to the labour market. It is significant in that, as Table 2.1 shows, considerable numbers of young people are both in full-time education *and* in employment. The expansion of employment opportunities can also be argued to have facilitated the expansion of post-16 education. Yet there is concern about the conditions of employment of young people. Many are employed in ways which are illegal, and there is a growing body of evidence that such employment may not accord with their welfare interests.

Article 32 of the United Nations Convention on the Rights of the Child clearly states the duty of governments to ensure that children doing work must be protected from conditions which are dangerous, which harm their health or interfere with their education. Current English law covering the employment of children dates back to 1933 (with a Scottish equivalent passed in 1937). The Employment Act of 1973 contained further provisions, but these have never been implemented (Lavalette 1994). Under British law, children should not be employed under the age of 13, and between 13 and 16 they should work only under a permit granted by a local authority. They should not start work before 7am or work after 7pm, while working on school days is restricted to two hours per day maximum (or up to a maximum of 17 hours per week for 11–15-year-olds, and 20 hours for those 15 and over). Paid work undertaken during school holidays can be for up to five hours a day for those between the ages of 11 and 15, and eight hours a day for those 15 and over (Lavalette et al., forthcoming).

The number of children and young people working while still in full-time education has, until recently, been little explored (Lavalette 1994). In a national survey, Baldwin found that around two-thirds of young people in the final year of compulsory schooling were working during term time (Balding 1991). Another study of pupils from a number of schools in Scotland and northern England reports that most school children now work, many do so illegally, and the jobs they do vary from the traditional part-time "youth jobs" such as delivery rounds, waiting jobs and baby-sitting, to shop work, and work on building sites and in garages (Lavalette et al., forthcoming). A fifth of this sample had started paid employment illegally, with some children reporting that they obtained their first job before the age of 10. Many were employed outside of the statutory allowed hours – some starting milk rounds as early as 5am – and nearly all of those reporting that they worked were unregistered and did not have the work permits required by law. More than a third started work before the permitted 7am and an even larger percentage worked after 7pm. Lavalette and colleagues argue that, by the last two years of compulsory schooling, most young people who work have graduated from "children's jobs" to jobs where "potentially they are in competition with adults in the labour market". Hourly wage rates are reported to be well below those recommended by the Low Pay Unit, the TUC and the Council of Europe (Lavalette et al. 1991). Students in colleges and at university are now also highly likely to engage in part-time employment.

What the growing "flexibility" of the labour market means is that fewer and fewer young people (mainly from working-class backgrounds) have been able to secure full-time jobs at minimum school-leaving age, while more and more children and young people have been able to secure part-time jobs while still at school. For those from more middle-class backgrounds, there has been an expansion of part-time work which provides them with a supplementary income during extended stays in further and higher education. This "flexibility" has also been enhanced by the abolition of the Wages Councils in August 1993. Following abolition, and based upon the New Earnings Survey 1993, Maclagan has calculated that there has been a drop of just under 1% in the earnings of young men under 18 years of age, and a 5.9% fall in the average wages of young women of the same age (Maclagan 1993). Not only are there fewer jobs for young people, but the wage rates they obtain have begun to decline. In all these changes in the structure of the youth labour market, it is largely working-class early school-leavers who have suffered. Those who might be argued to have benefited include those young people who choose to stay on in education beyond minimum school-leaving age. The size of this group increased markedly at the beginning of the 1990s. It is to the restructuration of the education system that we now turn.

Education reform, the education debate and the growth of post-16 education

The growth of youth unemployment, especially among young people, can be argued to have triggered a number of debates about both

45

the quality and suitability of mainstream educational provision and the willingness and ability of educational professionals to produce a workforce which is adequately educated and trained for the needs of a modern economy. A group of authors from the Centre for Contemporary Cultural Studies (CCCS) in Birmingham has provided a useful review of the disparate sources of these debates, from campaigns run by tabloid newspapers, to a series of Black Papers on Education emanating from New Right authors and industrialists (CCCS 1981). Doubts about whether education was sufficiently in tune with the needs and interests of industry were expressed long before the election of the first Thatcher Government in 1979. Starting with a series of Black Papers on education in the late 1960s and early 1970s, serious concern about educational standards was voiced by the Labour Prime Minister James Callaghan in his (in)famous Ruskin Speech in 1976. Education was accused of failing to give young people proper vocational education or training and of steering the best brains towards academia and the civil service, rather than areas in the national interest such as industry and commerce (CCCS 1981). Brown has argued that Callaghan's endorsement of points initially raised by New Right authors finally marked the death of one consensus and the growth of another (Brown 1988). Education, it was argued, no longer could be regarded as an end in itself nor as meeting an open-ended right to knowledge *per se*. Since 1976 a number of reforms in the education service mean that the knowledge (and skills) required to be produced in young people have been made increasingly accountable to the perceived needs of industry. By the time of the steep rises in unemployment in the early 1980s, the Thatcher administration was increasingly insistent upon vocational initiatives in schools and colleges (Dale 1985). These have included the development and expansion (and embedding or demise?) of the Technical and Vocational Educational Initiative (Inspectorate of Schools 1991), the development of Schools Industry Links and Business-Education Partnerships (CBI 1988), the expansion and reform of work experience programmes for 15–16-year-olds (National Curriculum Council 1991), and new forms of vocational education developed in partnership with industry and commerce (CBI 1988).

Despite these and other developments in vocational education, the most publicized arena of change in education policy during the Thatcher Governments came with the debates around the Education

Reform Act 1988, and its implementation since then. Paradoxically this Act seemed oblivious to the vocational initiatives of the 1970s and early 1980s (Coles 1988). In introducing the Bill before Parliament, however, the then Minister of Education and Science, Kenneth Baker, did make clear the government's intentions to make the education service less "producer dominated" and more accountable to the consumer. He made clear that this implied, not so much greater pupil choice, but "freeing schools and colleges to deliver the standards that *parents and employers* want" (quoted in Haviland 1988: 2, emphasis added). Education policy makers in the late 1980s and 1990s have been determined to switch the balance of interest, through changes in the control of education, away from professional educationalists (who were considered to have failed in their responsibilities to the wider community) and towards parents (who could be relied upon to insist upon standards) and industrialists (who were, it was argued, best placed to determine what sort of education and training was most required). This rebalancing of interests has been achieved through a number of initiatives introduced by the 1988 Act and set in train before it. These include the development of City Technology Colleges, the strengthening of the role of parent governors, the development of local management of schools and delegated budgets, and the encouragement and promotion of grant-maintained schools which opt out of local authority control (Chitty & Simon 1993, Maclure 1988, Simon 1988). Competition between schools and the nature of school funding were changed under reforms brought in under the Education Reform Act 1988. As a result, schools have a direct financial incentive in getting more and more students to stay in education for longer (Leonard 1988, Maclure 1988). With more than a £2,000 payment for each 16-year-old staying on at school, encouraging more to do so also saves teachers' jobs. Responsibility for the content of education has passed to central government through the introduction of the National Curriculum and central government-appointed bodies (such as the Schools Curriculum and Assessment Agency). The interests of industrialists were further highlighted by the government's acceptance and endorsement of "Education and Training Targets" drawn up by the Confederation of British Industry (CBI), as set out in *The skills revolution* (CBI 1990, Department of Education and Science, Department of Employment, Welsh Office 1991).

In all the debate about the impact of both "new vocationalism" and the Education Reform Act 1988, relatively little attention has been given to a third area of change which was to prove of critical importance in the restructuring of the school-to-work transition – the introduction of the General Certificate of Secondary Education (GCSE) examination for 16-year-olds in 1986. In part at least, this was introduced in order to bring together two systems of examination (the broadly academic GCE and the CSE which, prior to 1986, was targeted at students perceived to be less able). Yet the new examination was innovatory not only in bridging two examinations. It also introduced assessment through course work, completed during the final two years of compulsory schooling, as well as end-of-year examinations (Ainley 1991). This has proved to have had a marked impact upon the numbers of 16-year-olds obtaining moderate to good qualifications – and in raising the possibilities of them staying in full-time education beyond minimum school-leaving age. This has also been aided by an increase in the variety of post-16 courses available to them.

Gray, Jesson and Tranmer have attempted to examine some of the reasons behind the growth in participation rates in post-16 education. They examine a number of potential contributory causes including gender, ethnicity, social class background (measured both in terms of parental occupation and the educational qualifications attained by parents), the state of local labour markets, types of educational provision and changes in benefit entitlement (Gray et al. 1993). Reviewing evidence of the link between unemployment rates and post-16 participation in education, they indicate that, until the mid-1980s, the two rates seem to be inextricably linked. Yet, as unemployment rates began to fall in the late 1980s, education participation rates continued to rise. They report the impact of benefit changes as having only a limited measurable effect in influencing groups who may have previously left education at minimum school-leaving age to stay on for longer. Evidence of the impact of different types of education system is also reported to be inconclusive. Research undertaken earlier for the Department of Employment had reported that the introduction of one-year vocational courses had had some impact upon both increasing participation rates and diverting this group from subsequent unemployment (Sime et al. 1990). Gray et al. are less convinced that the evidence is yet conclusive, although they do comment that merely repeating fifth-year qualifications is less attractive and "efforts to increase the relevance and attractiveness of post-16 qualifications may well prove important in encouraging previously deterred young people to consider staying on" (Gray et al. 1993: 13).

Social class background has long been associated with both the attitudes young people have towards the value of education and their attractiveness to employers when they enter the labour market (Ashton et al. 1988). In reviewing the evidence from the YCS, Gray and his colleagues note that there is indeed an observable relationship, but that its relative importance diminishes when examination achievements are taken into account. Re-analyzing material from the Scottish school-leaver surveys between 1977 and 1987, Furlong also concluded that, while those from lower social classes did suffer most during the recession, when he controlled for the qualifications obtained at 16, young people from working-class families were only slightly more vulnerable than they had been a decade earlier (Furlong 1992). Qualifications at 16 have been significantly improved by the introduction of the GCSE examination in 1986 (DES-DfE Annual Statistics 1986–93). The analysis of the YCS also leads Gray and colleagues to a positive evaluation of some of the educational reforms of the mid-1980s. They accept that one impact of the GCSE reforms was that "by lifting the qualifications profile of the whole cohort it follows that . . . more young people will reach particular levels of attainment . . . and the overall proportion staying on will increase" (Gray et al. 1993: 13). So, while other factors may have had a marginal impact upon staying on rates, they conclude that "the single most important factor driving the decision to stay on is the level of qualifications at sixteen-plus" (Gray et al. 1993: 19). This seems to bear testimony to the fact that policy intervention in education may have had a marked effect upon the changing shape of youth transitions.

The three features of education reform we have described, together with changes in the youth labour market described in the previous section, provide the context in which we must understand the remarkable growth in post-16 education during the 1990s. During the late 1980s and 1990s, there has been a proliferation of different post-16 options within education. The pattern of choice for 16-year-olds is now much more complex than existed even as late as 1988 when the Educational Reform Act was passed by Parliament. In the mid-1990s, 16-year-olds and their parents have a choice of both the institutions young people can attend and an extended range of courses available in each institution. Table 2.2 is based on official statistics from the Department for Education and documents the patterns of change in the 1980s and early 1990s. Several features of this table deserve interpretation and comment. First, the numbers of 16-year-olds involved in full-time education nearly doubled between 1979 and 1992, with the largest expansion coming at the beginning of the 1990s. Secondly, although there has been some marked expansion in traditional academic studies (A and A/S levels), much more expansion has taken place in other sectors.

Table 2.2 Participation of 16-year-olds in education in England, 1979/80 to 1992/93 (% of all 16-year-olds in England).

	1979–80	1985–6	1989–90	1992–3
Full-time courses				
A and A/S levels				
Maintained schools	12.5	12.1	14.8	16.9
Sixth-form colleges	2.3	2.8	3.5	5.1
Tertiary colleges	–	0.6	1.4	1.8
Other maintained colleges	1.2	1.2	1.8	4.2
Independent schools	4.4	4.4	5.6	6.1
Total	20.4	21.1	27.5	32.5
BTEC national				
Maintained schools	–	–	–	0.7
Sixth-form colleges	–	–	–	0.2
Tertiary colleges	–	0.3	0.4	0.8
Other maintained colleges	1.8	3.0	2.9	5.3
Independent schools				
Total	1.8	3.3	3.4	6.1
All other courses				
Maintained schools				
Sixth-form colleges	1.0	1.4	1.7	2.4
Tertiary colleges	–	2.7	1.9	2.7
Other maintained colleges	8.2	8.8	9.5	16.4
Independent schools	0.9	0.9	0.9	0.8
Total	15.0	18.9	20.2	28.8
Total numbers (thousands)				
In full time education (FTE)	149	165.4	170.9	193.3
Population of 16-year-olds	396.4	376.3	325.7	284.7
% in FTE	37.6	44.0	51.7	67.9
% of 16-year-olds in part-time courses	21.4	19.9	18.8	9.5

Source: based on Department for Education 1993, table 1.

The table further shows that there has been more than a three-fold increase in students taking vocational BTEC national courses, although this still only commands a 6% market share of the age group. A more significant development has taken place in "other courses", which include both further GCSE courses and also other vocational courses often initially of only one year in duration. The latter include BTEC first diplomas, from which students can proceed to BTEC national diploma courses. This group also, however, includes diplomas and certificates of vocational education and, since 1992, General National Vocational Qualifications (GNVQs). Despite the growing numbers of young people opting to take these qualifications, there remains a doubt about their quality (Smithers 1993). Their introduction seems to have been an unexpected success, in terms of student take-up of the courses, although worries still exist about how they will be regarded by institutions of higher education and employers. Taking both these developments together, what is clear is that the expansion of post-16 education has included a significant increase in vocational education.

While the DfE data are for England alone, similar increases can be observed in other parts of the United Kingdom. *Regional Trends* for 1994 indicates that, by 1992–3, 76.8% of all 16-year-olds stayed on in education, while there was also some marked regional variation. In Northern Ireland, nearly nine out of ten (88.1%) continued their full-time education post-16, while Scotland and Wales reported staying-on rates of 77% and 75% respectively. There were also some variations within the regions of England, with Yorkshire and Humberside providing post-16 education participation rates of 69.1% compared to 80.5% in the South-East and 81.3% in the South-West (*Regional Trends* 1994).

At first sight this expansion of post-16 full-time education seems to be a success story. Increases in qualifications attained at 16 plus are resulting in higher participation rates in education after the age of 16, and increased qualifications have, in the past, been related to later success in the labour market. Ashford et al. are also guardedly enthusiastic about increases in post-16 participation rates and report that the better-qualified young people are embarking upon two-year post-16 courses, and that there is some evidence of the widening of the social class base of post-compulsory education. They also report that there is little evidence from the YCS of higher rates of participation being linked to higher drop-out or failure rates (Gray et al. 1993). Yet, an Audit Commission report on college courses suggests a less optimistic picture. One of the headline findings of the research, already referred to in Chapter 1 is that 150,000 young people per year (between 30% and 40% of those starting a full-time post-16 course) leave "without achieving what the course was designed for, either through leaving early or through failure in the relevant examination and assessment" (Audit Commission & OFSTED 1993: 24). The Audit Commission report examined the circumstances in which the drop-out from courses was most likely to occur and indicated that this was most likely when young people with relatively few 16+ qualifications are admitted to courses. Such recruitment, they report, may be either inappropriate selection by college authorities, or result in young people themselves judging that they had made the wrong choice of course and subsequently leaving. It should be remembered that, under the new funding arrangements for schools and colleges, each institution has a direct financial incentive to recruit. The Audit Commission report leaves serious doubts as to whether young people are receiving adequate information, guidance and advice about their choices of education and training careers at the age of 16. Youth Cohort Study data confirm that the growth in the proportion of the age group staying in full-time education at 16 has been at the expense of early entrants to the labour market, either into YT or employment outside of YT. It is notable too that there are sex differences in the ways in which "extended transitions" have developed. Between 1984 and 1991, young men's participation in education increased from 31% to 53%, whereas young women's increased from 42% to 64%.

The precarious transition without benefit of a safety net

In 1982, Roberts reports that over a quarter (27.6%) of young people between the ages of 16 and 18 were unemployed. At that time they were entitled to receive Supplementary Benefit, Housing Benefit and a number of other means to provide them with the wherewithal to live. With the implementation of the Fowler social security reforms introduced by the Social Security Acts of 1986 and 1988, young people were no longer eligible to claim the replacement for Supplementary Benefit (Income Support). Flat Rate Grants for the purchase of essential items had been replaced by the Social Fund (for which most young people would be unlikely to qualify as a high priority group), and other benefit entitlements had also been withdrawn. The withdrawal of the entitlement to Income Support (IS) was meant to be commensurate with the government guarantee that all young people not in employment or full-time education should be given a place of Youth Training for which they would be given a training allowance (albeit at the time of a rate for 16-year-olds of only £29.50 per week). To all intents and purposes this withdrawal of entitlement defined away unemployment among 16–18-year-olds at a stroke, but the problems of unemployed young people of this age group have not disappeared.

The Unemployment Unit has made an attempt to calculate the numbers of unemployed according to the rules in operation in 1979 and to estimate the numbers of young people without work and not on training schemes. In July 1993, it estimated that there were 95,600 16- and 17-year-olds unemployed. Of these, 67,505 had no job, no training and no benefits. However, July traditionally has the lowest rates of unemployment. The October 1992 estimate of the Unemployment Unit for the same age group was 124,700, and in May 1994 the chairman of the Conservative Party, Sir Norman Fowler, admitted to a European election press conference that 76,000 school-leavers had slipped through the training and benefits safety net (*Independent* 1 June 1994).

These figures from the Unemployment Unit on unemployment among this age group are broadly in line with the Department of Employment Labour Force Surveys estimates. The 1992 survey estimated that 125,000 16–17-year-olds were unemployed according to internationally agreed definitions of unemployment, just short of 10% of the age group. Despite ineligibility for the main benefit (IS), there are now two separate means through which some young 16–18-year-olds can receive benefits. After the summer vacation following the end of compulsory schooling, if they cannot be offered a place on Youth Training, they may be entitled to a "bridging allowance" for eight weeks. Some young people under the age of 18 can also apply for "severe hardship payments" if the Benefits Agency accepts that they are estranged from their parents and the training guarantee is not being met. In the mid-1990s, as young people became more aware of these special payments, applications for them increased significantly. The number of young people applying for Severe Hardship Allowances increased by 23% in 1993–4 to 141,644, and the number awarded the allowance also rose by 30%, to 123,757, a success rate of 87%. Yet there were signs that the Treasury was worried about this drift of public expenditure upwards (£40 million per year in 1993) and intended to tighten the criteria through which young people are eligible for such benefit (*Guardian* 2 June 1994). Unemployment among 16–24-year-olds is considerably higher than for other age groups. The Unemployment Unit estimates for July 1993 indicated that 875,900 young people in this 16–24 age group (16.7% of the total) were unemployed. This represents an almost doubling of the unemployment of this age group since 1989 and approaching the 19% figure at the height of recession in 1985. Despite changes in education, training, the youth labour market and social security provision, therefore, youth unemployment has not gone away.

Winners and losers and the threat to young people's rights

Who, then, are the winners and losers from these changes in education and the labour market? The losers are easier to identify than the winners. What is clear is that the school-to-work transition has become hardest for those who, for a variety of reasons do not do well during compulsory schooling and leave with few or no qualifications. Some of these may be young people who were disillusioned with schooling, perhaps irregularly attended, and perhaps saw little value in school qualifications. Truancy league tables are to be introduced to allow parents to pin-point schools which are more or less successful in inspiring interest, involvement and attendance. Yet it is too easy to write off a lack of educational qualifications as the result of individual idleness, truancy or lack of ability. Carlen has argued that there is much pain, hurt, suffering and humiliation around "failure" and "exclusion" (Carlen et al. 1992). Exclusions from school have increased rapidly since the introduction of school qualification league tables in which each school is competing to impress with success in attaining qualifications rather than adding educational value. Furthermore, those who start their post-16 careers with the most severe disadvantages may do so because of a special educational need and/or being educated in a special school because of a disability. The unqualified will have least chance of obtaining employment, least chance of being recruited to a YT place with a good chance of employment, and will be most likely to suffer unemployment with no benefit.

The winners include those who take advantage of educational reform, stay in education for longer with a variety of different courses and institutions to choose from, and have better prospects of proceeding to higher education at the age of 18. There are some signs that these are no longer only the sons and daughters of professional and managerial workers, and that the expansion of further and higher education has finally widened access to social class and ethnic groups previously excluded from educational opportunities (UCCA statistics, various). But graduate unemployment is considerable, and rising. As with the displacement of youth jobs into training schemes, it is too early to tell whether this group may become the next generation of highly qualified, older, wiser, but disillusioned unemployed.

One of the main transitions of youth is that from full-time education to employment. Youth transitions involve difficult and dangerous choices between following one career option and another. Given this, young people need to have access to knowledge, guidance, advice and support if they are to avoid making inappropriate career choices. Until the 1990s, the Careers Service was firmly located within local authority education departments and prided itself on being an "honest broker" in offering – through professionally trained, publicly accountable, careers officers – impartial information, help and guidance, about *all* options in education, training or employment (Chubb 1988). In the 1990s, under the Employment Act 1993, the Careers Service was manoeuvred into the hands of Training and Enterprise Councils (TECs) – or in Scotland, Local Enterprise Councils (LECS) – and, in some parts of the country, is being "market tested", before being privatized and contracted with private companies. When under the ownership and control of local education authorities, the Careers Service was accountable to local councillors, with questions about the running of the service made in subcommittee meetings and reported by the local press. TEC boards, on the other hand, are appointees, and the board is required only to submit an annual report to a public meeting on all spheres of its activity. The local accountability of Careers Services, therefore, has been considerably diminished. There is clearly a continued need for impartial guidance and advice on the myriad of complex career choices now facing young people. If a young person leaves school in the *mistaken* belief that a training programme will lead to work, or conversely, if they stay on and take a course of education in some *mistaken* belief that this will lead to a secure job, then, where they act on *mistaken* beliefs, they suffer severe welfare harm as a result. Yet, in the reforms described above, the balance of powers between the providers of education, industry, young people and their parents has substantially changed. The net gainers are local industrialists and central government. But where are the safeguards that the rights and needs of young people will not be further eroded? The rights to *impartial* knowledge, education, guidance and advice about the implications of different and competing career choices is, therefore, one element which is essential to the welfare of young people.

National policy change, can also be seen to have eroded young people's rights to, and at, work. Restrictions on the working hours of young people have been abandoned, as have restrictions on the conditions in which they work. The abolition of Wages Councils has been argued to be an attempt to price the low paid, among whom the young figure, back into work. Yet, as a result, it has reduced the possibility of young people earning a wage which would afford them economic independency of their parents. The "wages" of those on training schemes have not been upgraded in line with either inflation or average wage rates. Social security support for young people who are unemployed has either been withdrawn or reduced; Income Support has been withdrawn from (nearly all) 16–17-year-olds, and new and reduced rates have been introduced for young people between the ages of 18 and 25. All this has fundamentally transformed the connection of young people to the labour market and placed more and more responsibilities upon families to give economic support to young people undertaking ever more extended transitions. It goes without saying that the most fundamental threat to young people's welfare and their rights lies in the absence of jobs and the fear of unemployment, which, as we approach the twenty-first century, still haunts the welfare of young careers.

Chapter Three

The re-structuration of youth: family structure and family relationships

In the last chapter we explored the changing nature of the school-to-work transition. It was argued that changes in the labour market and education mean that, in the 1990s, more and more young people are economically dependent upon their families for longer periods of time. Families are not, however, homogeneous and static repositories into which turbulent social change can be poured without strain, anxiety, resistance or confusion. Families are arenas of private dramas, complex negotiations between genders and generations, and conflicts of interest. And these private spheres have been subject to considerable change, public debate and legislative regulation in the last two decades as politicians, political and moral commentators, social scientists and family members have attempted to come to terms with changing patterns of family roles and responsibilities. While some authors have argued that the state should do all in its power to encourage a return to traditional models of family responsibilities (Dennis & Erdos 1992, Major 1993, Murray 1990), Finch & Mason have suggested that it is "not enough simply to assume that the family as a social institution is ready, willing and able to shoulder the burden of supporting its members who cannot fully care for themselves, either practically or financially" (Finch & Mason 1993: 10). They argue that it is difficult to draw a line between what families can and should do to meet the needs of members, and what the state must do in supporting its citizens. This is a recurring theme throughout this book.

Many of the fundamental mistakes about family policy and young people can be laid at the door of a mistaken conflation of family (or household) *structures* and family *relationships*. In this chapter, a distinction will be made between family structure, by which is meant the number of adults, children and young people living within a single household and the status relationship between them, and family relationships, which refer to the nature and quality of interactions between parents and offspring. The conflation of structure and relationship has resulted in lone-parent families being scapegoated by some writers and politicians, without any real consideration of either the cause of lone parenthood, or the quality of relationship between parent and child (Braid 1993, Murray 1990). In similar fashion, two-parent families have received favourable comment, without any consideration of the nature and quality of relationship between parents, the impact of the relationship between parents on the parent–child relationship, or the role of the (particularly male) parent with the child (Dennis & Erdos 1992). As Jones has pointed out, some two-parent families have fathers who work away from home (often for months at a time), while in some others one parent is incapacitated either by chronic illness or alcoholism and, therefore, rarely contributes positively to family life (Jones 1994). On the other hand, as her research indicates, some who appear in statistics based on questionnaire surveys as lone parents are found, when they are followed up, to have several members of either the extended family or close friends in support of the mother. What this chapter will attempt to describe is the current state of knowledge about who does what in families. Who does what about a child's or young person's health, ill-health or welfare? Who is the gatekeeper to statutory medical support? When, and under what circumstances, do young people take responsibility for what is happening and what can be done to their own bodies? Who attempts to control and discipline young people's behaviour? How do young people respond? How, and in what ways, are parents influential in determining young people's educational and occupational careers? And does the increasing likelihood of their living with their parents for longer periods of time (extended transitions) mean that these patterns of responsibility, constraint and control are less assured, fractious, or more brittle? Are parental power and control more likely to be ignored or resisted, or result in family breakdown? While much of the media attention has been focused on family structure, many of the critical questions can be seen to rest on family relationships. This remains a vital but under-explored area of social research. Despite the, often acrimonious and uninformed, nature of the debate about the family and the welfare of young people, few would dispute that family structure and family relationships have been subject to rapid social change in the last two decades, and that the nature and extent of these changes have been influential in re-shaping the welfare environment in which young people grow up. It is with changes in family structures that we begin the discussion.

Changes in family structures

While it is relatively straightforward to describe changes in family structures, the simple descriptions sometimes disguise complex patterns of development. So, for instance, demographic statistics can tell us that the number of lone-parent families has more than doubled from 570,000 in 1971 to 1,270,000 in 1991 (Burghes 1994). Since the 1960s there has been a fourfold increase in the number of divorces. Remarriages have also increased more than threefold, from just short of 37,000 in 1961 to 148,000 in 1991. In static, cross-sectional terms, 8 per cent of children and young people now live in "reconstituted" families with a step-parent, although, as we will see, this underestimates the proportion of young people who will experi-ence the divorce and/or remarriage of their parents before they reach adulthood. There has also been a dramatic increase in the numbers of "single parents" – approaching a fivefold increase in the number of single (never married) parents (Burghes 1994, Haskey 1990, 1991, 1992, 1993, 1994). These simple facts describe both widespread and rapid social change. On the basis of a special set of questions intro-duced by the Office of Population Census and Surveys (OPCS) and the General Household Survey 1990–2, Haskey has estimated the distri-bution of different types of families containing dependent children (Haskey 1994). This is summarized in Table 3.1. Yet none of the sim-ple factual statements, nor the implications of the table, can be under-stood without considerable qualification being made to both the definition of family types and what these might mean for the life cir-cumstances of young people living in families.

At its simplest, one could conclude from this table that three-quarters of children and young people are living with their biological

Table 3.1 Distribution of families with dependent children by "family type" 1990–1992.

	% of all families	Mean number of children per family	% of children in family type
All couple families with natural children only	75.6	1.9	75.5
Married couples	71.2	1.9	72.8
Cohabiting couples	3.5	1.5	2.7
All one parent families	**18.6**	**1.8**	**16.6**
Lone mother families	16.6	1.7	14.8
Lone father families	2.0	1.6	1.8
Married couple (MC) step families			
Total MC step families	4.6	2.3	5.6
Natural mother	3.4	2.1	3.9
Natural father	0.9	2.4	1.1
Step mother and step father	0.3	0.6	0.6
Cohabiting couple step families			
All cohabiting step families	2.1	2.2	2.2
Natural mother	1.6	1.9	1.6
Natural father	0.3	1.8	0.3
Step mother and step father	0.1	3.2	0.3

Source: based on Haskey 1994, table 1.

parents, one in six (16.6%) are living in lone-parent families, while around 8% are living in reconstituted families with a parent who has either remarried or is cohabiting. Yet, two important conceptual points need to be borne in mind. First, much of the literature on family structures describes static structures. Much of the survey data, such as those on which Table 3.1 is based, describe the distribution of family structures at one moment in time. Many families represented within these statistics contain young parents and children who are likely to experience a change in their family circumstances as both the parent and child get older. So, for instance, a child who is currently in the table as a young child living with a lone parent may experience the cohabitation and later marriage of its parent (either to the child's natural parent or someone else), a partnership breakdown and/or divorce, the re-partnering of its parent and perhaps a later remarriage. All this may take place before the child reaches adulthood. A number of researchers have attempted to reinterpret the static picture of family types, by projecting on to the data a series of trends in fam-

ily development, which allow us to predict what will h;
families given the passage of time. After doing this, Ha
that, by the age of 16, nearly a quarter of young p(
experienced the divorce of their parents and many o
in reconstituted families. More startlingly, Kiernan & Wicks have estimated that, given current trends in divorce and lone parenthood, by
the end of the century, the percentage of young people being brought
up according to the "conventional pattern" of living with both their
married biological parents until they are grown up will have fallen to
as low as 50% (Kiernan & Wicks 1990).

Secondly, and following from this, we must think of family consti-
tution and reconstitution as a process rather than as simply changes in
structure. All family relationships involve the negotiation and renegotiation of roles and responsibilities, freedoms and duties, and patterns of care and control. When young people experience the breakup and/or reconstitution of their families, it is now widely recognized
that this is best thought of as a complex set of processes taking place
over a considerable time, rather than as a simple or discrete event.
When children and young people experience the separation and
divorce of their parents, this may have wide-ranging consequences on
where they live, the schools they attend, and their material and emotional circumstances. It is, furthermore, part of a complex and elon-
gated process which may start with family disharmony, result in lone
parenthood and may involve (sooner or later) becoming part of a
step-parent family involving new relationships with a step-parent and
stepbrothers or -sisters. Chase-Lansdale & Hetherington, based on
research undertaken in the United States, suggest that the impact of
divorce on children often takes two or more years to emerge and the
adjustment to this and any subsequent stepfamily may take much
longer than adjustment to the divorce itself (Chase-Lansdale &
Hetherington 1990).

Family structure and material circumstances

Much of our knowledge about the different material circumstances
of different family types is based on work conducted in the late 1980s
by Bradshaw & Millar. They have argued that a close examination of
different types reveals that they differ according to the average age of
parents and children, and, consequent upon that, their main source,
and level, of income (Bradshaw & Millar 1991). They have estimated

61

that the average age of *single* parents is 24 and that they have on average 1.4 children, with in six out of ten cases, a child under the age of 5. Because single parents are looking after a child under school age, they are also highly likely to be dependent upon Income Support as their main source of income. Nine out of ten such families were on Income Support in 1986 (Bradshaw & Millar 1991, Burghes 1994). As Bradshaw & Millar have argued, the main problem such families face is balancing the wish to be good parents with being breadwinners. Most single parents wish to work but few can do so because of the cost of nursery places and the need to care for pre-school children. Based on Bradshaw & Millar's research, Burghes estimates that 18% of single parents are also still living in the parental home. Of the rest, the vast majority (80%) are living in local authority accommodation (Burghes 1994). Single parents are, therefore, young, poor and very dependent upon state support which is perhaps why they have become the "bogeywoman" of Britain in the early 1990s (Braid 1993).

Separated or divorced lone mothers, on the other hand, are much more likely to be older. Three-quarters of divorced mothers are between the ages of 30 and 44, while 70% of separated mothers are between 25 and 39. They are likely to have larger families than single-parent families, with an average number of 1.9 children. More than half (58%) of divorced mothers, and 45% of separated mothers, have children over the age of 10. Separated and divorced mothers also share other characteristics regarding the financial and housing circumstances in which they live. Whereas, before 1992, few single parents received regular maintenance payments (the General Household Survey reported in 1989 that only 13% did so), around half of the divorced mothers, and around a third of separated mothers, received maintenance payments (Bradshaw & Millar 1991, Burghes 1993, General Household Survey 1989). Divorced and separated parents are much more likely to be in employment than single mothers. Just over half of the divorced mothers had jobs; three out of ten of them full-time paid work. Many were in employment before they became divorced, although four out of ten stopped work when they became lone parents (Bradshaw & Millar 1991). This means they were better off than single parents but still considerably less well off than those living in two-parent families.

The number of one-parent families headed by a father almost doubled in the 1970s and 1980s, reaching 130,000 in 1989 (Burghes 1993). Lone-father families are likely to have both older parents and older children. One-quarter of male lone-parent families are the result of bereavement rather than separation or divorce. Fathers are more likely to be in their late 30s or 40s and nearly one in eight of lone-father families is composed of a father and a child over 10. Almost half of such families (48%) live in owner-occupied houses and six out of ten fathers in these families are in full-time work. In brief, lone-parent families come about for a variety of different reasons and experience a range of different material circumstances (Popay & Jones 1990). Both these sets of factors can be seen to be important in understanding the ways in which young people's lives are affected by changes in family structure.

A number of attempts have been made to examine the impact of living in different family structures on the welfare of children and the approaches young people make to the main transitions of youth. Some of the material is now rather dated as it is based on large-scale cohort studies which started in the 1940s and late 1950s, when the stigma of illegitimate birth and divorce was much greater than it was in the 1980s and early 1990s (Crellin et al. 1971). Elliott & Richards suggest that the behaviour of young people at the age of 16 is influenced by the experience of divorce but that these differences can be seen to have been occurring before the divorce itself (Elliott & Richards 1991a). They focus on two measures: "disruptive behaviour" and children and young people being "unhappy and worried". They report being "unhappy and worried" as intensified by early marital disruption (before the child was between 7 and 11 years of age). There is some suggestion that boys and girls respond in different ways. The data suggest that girls are more likely to persist in being "unhappy and worried" into their teenage years, while boys show more immediate signs of disruptive behaviour. Elliott & Richards further report that there are observed differences in the educational attainments of children living with divorced parents, with lower reported scores on test of mathematical and reading ability at both the ages of 11 and 16. But they add that these differences were also observed at the age of 7 when the children's families were still intact (Elliott & Richards 1991b). Ferri, in an earlier study, claimed that differences in academic achievements at 7 and 11 disappeared once an allowance had been made for two correlated factors – income and class background (Ferri 1984). Later studies by Maclean & Wadsworth, whose analysis tried to control for social class, and Kuh & Maclean, who controlled for the potential influence of a mother's education, do, however, claim an influence of separation and divorce on the qualifications young people obtain (Kuh & Maclean 1990, Maclean & Wadsworth 1988). Young people who had experienced the separation or divorce of the parents were found to have a reduced chance of obtaining school qualifications and an increased chance of being unemployed at the age of 18. Wadsworth & Maclean further indicate that young people from separated families in which the father was in a manual occupation were likely to have jobs with a lower income than their contemporaries from other types of families (Wadsworth & Maclean 1986). Elliott & Richards also suggest that young people with separated or divorced parents were less likely to get a university qualification (Elliott & Richards 1991b). It is important, interesting and noteworthy that all the studies reported above indicate that there are few, if any, significant differences between the performance and behaviour of young people brought up in lone families which are caused by bereavement, compared to intact families. Despite the obvious traumas of bereavement, and the likely changes in the material circumstances the family must face, young people experiencing the death of a parent seem to recover much better than those experiencing the divorce or separation of parents. All the studies based on NCDS data report that children from families experiencing bereavement tend to mirror the behaviour of young people from intact families rather than that of those in other lone-parent families (Burghes 1993). The studies reported above suggest that there is some room for concern about trends in family structure. There is a growth in the number of young people being brought up in families in which they will experience divorce, being brought up by lone parents, and joining reconstituted families. The evidence indicates that this means that they will suffer adverse material and emotional circumstances and that, as a result, their educational performance and school qualifications may suffer. Given this, it is also difficult to avoid the conclusion that these changes in family structure may also adversely affect youth transitions.

Family structure and youth transitions

The most comprehensive study of the impact of family disruption on youth transitions has been undertaken by Kiernan (Kiernan 1992). As in the case of the studies quoted above, this is based on the experience of children growing up in the 1960s and 1970s. NCDS data from the cohort born in 1958 and surveyed as they reached the ages of 16 and 22 are limited in the sense that, as this group reached minimum school-leaving age, the unemployment rate stood at only 5%. Young people approaching school-leaving age in the 1990s face much higher rates of unemployment and, as we saw in the last chapter, part of the response to this has been a growing tendency to stay in education for longer periods of time. The NCDS data are useful, however, in point- ing to the different experiences of transitions of young people brought up in different types of family structure. Kiernan reports that, by the time the NCDS cohort born in 1958 reached the age of 18, the vast majority (88%) were still members of intact families. Six per cent were in lone-mother families, 4% were in stepfamilies and less than 2% were in lone-father families. Kiernan examined a number of different transitions, including leaving school, starting work, leaving home, getting married and becoming a parent. She reports first, that young people from families which had experienced marital break- down are more likely to leave school at the age of 16. She expresses "likelihood" in terms of "odds" when comparing the different family types with the average of young people from "intact" two-parent families. Boys from stepfamilies were nearly twice as likely (1.8) to leave school at 16, closely followed by boys from lone-mother fami- lies (1.6). Girls from all families were less likely to leave school at 16, but girls from lone-mother families did leave more often with the odds of their doing so being 1.3 compared to girls from intact two- parent families. In a more recent, though smaller-scale, study of young people drawn from a single West London borough and con- ducted in the late 1980s, Brannen and colleagues report similar dif- ferences, although with a predictably higher base in the sense that all young people were more likely to stay on in education at the age of 16. In this more recent study, the vast majority (84%) planned to stay in education at minimum school-leaving age. Young people living with lone mothers were slightly less likely to plan to do so (78%), those living with stepfathers less likely again (72%), and those living in other arrangements, including living with stepmothers (but also including other relatives), the least likely (56%) to stay on in education at the age of 16 (Brannen et al. 1994).

Secondly, Kiernan examined the likelihood of leaving home by the age of 18, comparing young people living in different family types. Girls appeared more likely to leave home "early" if they had experienced any form of family disruption and especially so if they had experienced parental marital breakdown. Boys too followed this pattern, with the exception of those living with lone mothers. In a study of young people in Scotland, Jones has distinguished between positive and negative reasons for leaving home. The positive reasons she identified are described as "traditional" and "socially legitimate", in that they included leaving home to marry, to continue education, or pursue an occupational career. Negative reasons tended to be "push factors" and included friction at home, being told to leave, poor or inadequate accommodation, or moving away from an area with no job prospects without any definite job to go to elsewhere (Jones 1993a). We will return to this study in more detail later in the chapter. Kiernan distinguishes between a similar set of positive and negative reasons for leaving and relates these to a wide range of transitions. She reports that, by the time the NCDS cohort had reached the age of 23, nine out of ten of the cohort had left the parental home for positive reasons. Yet young women from families involving step-parents, and young men who had experienced family disruption (with the notable exception of those living with lone mothers), were much more likely to have left for negative reasons, mainly because of family friction with parents or step-parents. Jones reports a similar pattern of response to step-parents, commenting that sometimes the natural parent sided with the step-parent in a way in which the young person regarded as an act both of betrayal and rejection (Jones 1993a).

Thirdly, Kiernan reports on the relationship between living in different family types and young people's transitions to new partnerships, marriage and having children of their own. The data she analyzed suggest that young people who experience the divorce of their parents, and young people living with step-parents, are more likely to start partnerships, marry and have children at an earlier age than young people in other family types. Young women, especially, where they had experienced divorce or separation of their parents, were much more likely to establish partnerships in their teens, although this was not true of daughters of women who had suffered bereavement. Women from stepfamilies reconstituted after divorce illustrated what Kiernan described as an "intriguing" propensity to *marry* at an early age, with the odds that they would do so as 3.6 times more than women from intact families (Kiernan 1992). Kuh & Maclean further report that, in the cohort they studied, by the age of 36, women whose parents had been divorced were also likely to have been teenage brides, to have been divorced themselves, and twice as likely to have been married more than once than women from intact families (Kuh & Maclean 1990). In Kiernan's study, young men who had experienced step-parent families were also more than twice as likely to have developed their first partnerships before the age of 20 than young men from intact families. They were also more likely to be married by the age of 21 and be fathers by the age of 23. Yet for those who had experienced other patterns of family disruption, especially those brought up with lone mothers, there was no noticeable difference in the age at which they started their own families compared to those brought up with both natural parents (Kiernan 1992). On the basis of this evidence, one has to conclude that the experience of family disruption does impact upon youth transitions, with young people who experience the divorce of their parents more likely to leave home earlier, start partnerships and marry earlier, and have children themselves at an earlier stage in their life course than young people brought up in intact families. It should also be remembered that Kiernan & Wicks predict that the number of young people brought up in such circumstances is rising dramatically (Kiernan & Wicks 1990). Whether they will all follow the pattern of attempting earlier transitions, as set in the 1970s, remains to be seen. The worry remains that while most young people now experience extended transitions, young people from families which have experienced divorce and reconstitutions may leave education and their family at an early stage, with potentially perilous consequences.

Most of the studies reported above rely upon a comparison of the average behaviours of young people living in different types of family structure. Yet there are obvious problems in reaching firm conclusions based upon such comparisons (Burghes 1994). One of the most basic problems faced when using family classifications is that the classificatory system treats a family structure as unitary and static, rather than allowing for a description or understanding of the dynamic processes of family life. As we have already argued, simple classifications allow no examination of the type of relationship a parent and child may experience throughout the process of growing up, or of how the quality of relationships may change over time. Nor do such studies allow for an examination of a variable outcome from each family type or the circumstances in which this might occur. Qualitative research on family relationships is much more likely to be able to unravel and describe such issues. So, for instance, in her study of young people and their housing careers, Jones indicates that, while step-parenting is a common structural feature of young people leaving home "prematurely", in some circumstances some step-parents are able to offer positive help and support (Jones 1994). She also points to the use and influence of wider kinship networks (aunts and uncles, brothers and sisters, for instance), as young people move away from the parental home. Finch & Mason have also pointed to the importance of wider kinship groupings. Indeed, they argue that what makes families distinct social institutions are the ways in which family members fulfil social obligations by offering assistance and material support without thought for personal gain (Finch & Mason 1993). While much of this is open to constant negotiation and re-negotiation, there are structural norms and expectations which continue to set parameters which keep these obligations in place. It is to the negotiation of family relationships within structural norms that we now turn.

Young people and family relationships

There have been a number of qualitative studies of family relationships concerning young people and their parents in recent years (Allatt & Yeandle 1992, Brannen et al. 1994, Finch 1989, Finch & Mason 1993, Hutson & Jenkins 1987, Jones & Gilliland 1993, Jones 1994, Wallace 1987). Some of these have focused on specific types of relationship or on families which face changing and difficult circumstances, such as unemployment (Hutson & Jenkins 1987, Wallace 1987). The study by Brannen and her colleagues has as its main focus family relationships and health, but within this it usefully examines a range of issues concerning the care and control parents exercise over their teenage children, together with the ways in which young people negotiate freedom and independence. The study is based on a sample drawn from one local authority in West London, but it does include households where the young people attend both private and state schools, and covers a range of different family types and ethnic backgrounds. The data on which the study draws are both from a large representative sample of more than 800 young people who supplied data via a questionnaire, and 142 in-depth interviews with household members based on a subsample of the initial questionnaire survey. While the study reports on different patterns of care and control, it also examines the ways in which these are negotiated. The authors argue that

> a major theme common to paternal and maternal narratives is the struggle of young people towards some notion of independent adulthood, on the one hand, and parents' concern to control and shape this process on the other. An underlying fear is that parents will not get the balance between care and control right, and will so alienate their sons and daughters that they will remove themselves altogether from parental control. In their response to this fear, and in many other aspects of the general change of parenting in the teenage years, mothers and fathers differ. (Brannen et al. 1994: 66)

This important and crucial last point is a useful antidote to treating the family as a unitary structure, rather than focusing on the different ways in which different members of a family are involved in different relationships of care and control. The traditional division of responsibility assumed in dual-parent families has often been described as one in which mothers "care" and fathers "control" (Parsons 1942). Much of this is based on the assumption that mothers were first and foremost parents, while fathers were predominantly breadwinners, playing a more important role outside of the family and providing a bridge between the private world of families and the public world of the economy and capitalism (Zaretsky 1976). Yet, in the 1990s most mothers of teenagers undertake paid work; in the study by Brannen et al. more than half of them were in full-time work. Despite this, nearly all of the mothers (98%) reported that they attempted to fit their employment around their family responsibilities, whereas most fathers (74%) described this the other way round as family responsibilities being fitted around their job. Nor were gender roles within families confined to employment commitments. Mothers, much more than fathers, were knowledgeable about their teenager's friends and what they did when they were not at home. It was mothers and not fathers who were, therefore, in a better position to attempt to control young people's behaviour and indeed they attempted to do so. So, for instance, it was mothers who tried to regulate and enforce rules about when their sons or daughters went out, how often this was, the time they should return home, and for how long they did homework, as well as other sets of behaviour concerning diet, health and health-promoting activity. It is mothers, therefore, who play the vital role in *both* the care *and* control of teenage children (Brannen et al. 1994).

Fathers, on the other hand, did have high opinions about their relationships with teenagers and positive views about teenagers as a group. They more often claimed to be closer to their son or daughter than their wife was, that their offspring took after them in terms of family characteristics, and that their teenager got on better with them than with their mother. Those fathers born in the United Kingdom were particularly reported as determined that they would be better fathers than their fathers had been to them and less hierarchical and distant in their dealings with their children. Mothers laid great store by communicating with their sons and daughters and building relationships of trust so that young people could confide in them and discuss with them their worries and anxieties. Parents, particularly those of white UK descendants, were reported as trading openness for freedom, in the hope that, in return for being given greater responsibilities and freedoms, young people would let them know where they were when they were not at home, with whom they associated, and what they did. Despite the self-confidence of fathers, however, it was mothers who were most named by teenagers as the adult with whom they got on best (Brannen et al. 1994).

Again it was mothers, rather than fathers, who were also key actors in what Brannen et al. term an individual's "illness career". They had knowledge of children's health history, were highly sensitive in first noticing signs of illness, and in prompting medical attention. Mothers often prescribed home remedies and were instrumental in either sending their son or daughter to the doctor, or taking them themselves. In the majority of cases (54%) it was still mothers, rather than young people themselves, who made appointments with general practitioners. The study indicates that between the ages of 15 and 16, young people begin to go to see their GPs on their own, rather than with their parent (predominantly mothers), although by the age of 16 it is young men rather than young women who are more likely to go alone. There were surprisingly few young people in this research who went to the doctor's without the knowledge of their parents. Only two young white women had decided to obtain the contraceptive pill from their GP without their parents' knowledge, and only a few cases were cited where young people consulted their GP without the knowledge, or against the wishes, of parents. Fathers had very little involvement in health matters and this was limited to "exceptional circumstances". Indeed, many had difficulty in even recalling any illnesses their teenagers had had (Brannen et al. 1994).

There were gender differences also in the sort of control parents attempted to have over young women and young men. Sons and daughters had different battlegrounds on which rules of behaviour were fought. Perhaps predictably, it was young women whose parents were most vigilant, especially about the frequency they were allowed to go out, the times they should return, and about drinking alcohol. Young men were restricted more in terms of smoking and doing homework. There were also differences between different ethnic groups in terms of the amount of control of behaviour and the areas where control was most likely to be exercised. Asian families proved to be the most strict and especially so with regard to smoking, drinking alcohol and going out. It was young people in white families who experienced the least strict enforcement of rules, and especially with regard to going out (Brannen et al. 1994).

Like other surveys, Brannen et al. report that a variety of different drugs are widely available, but that young people largely confine their drug use to cannabis. They report that, while nearly half of the 16-year-olds in their survey had been offered drugs, around one in five had taken cannabis. Many more of those attending private schools had been offered drugs than those in state schools and, despite drug use being an expellable offence in most private schools, nearly a third (29%) of 16-year-olds educated there reported taking cannabis. Hallucinogenic and hard drugs (including heroin and cocaine) were also more widely used in private schools, but they accounted for less than one in ten of those surveyed. This is broadly in line with other findings on drug use among young people (Plant & Plant 1992). Parents remain worried by the use of drugs despite the fact that many of them

71

were themselves brought up in an era when they would be likely to be exposed to widespread availability and a knowledge of the relative lack of danger associated with recreational drugs such as cannabis. In Brannen et al.'s study only one father and one mother approved of its use although ten parents admitted having used it themselves. Just over half of the young people said they were influenced by their parents' attitudes to drugs. Merchant & MacDonald have studied the use of Ecstasy among older groups of young people. While they are unable to offer reliable statistical estimates of its use, it is reported as widespread among those involved in rave culture, with some young people walking to school or work and skipping meals in order to finance weekend raves (Merchant & MacDonald 1994).

Food and diet were also important areas of negotiation between young people and their parents, with different patterns evolving in different families. The study by Brannen and her colleagues goes some way in denting the myth of "Bisto" families in which family meals are a major site of family unity and interaction. Many parents still clung to the importance of family meals, with just over half regarding them as important, although only a quarter of teenagers shared this view. Just over four out of ten families studied (42%) ate at least one meal together on most days and thought this pattern an important aspect of family life. This was more likely to be the case in Asian families, although several white middle-class families, including some stepfamilies shared this pattern and the belief in its importance. On the other hand, a third of young people only rarely ate as a family group. No matter what the pattern of eating, however, it was predominantly the mother who was responsible for food and diet.

Patterns of eating proved to be an important area in which parents and young people negotiated and renegotiated family roles. Indeed, these patterns can be read as symbolic of more general patterns of care and control, dependence and independence. In several of the families studied (14 out of 62), young people appeared to have got the upper hand. Brannen et al. describe four different patterns. The group described as the "resisters" either would not eat with their families or insisted on eating different food which they prepared themselves. Interestingly, all these were young women from middle-class backgrounds who were high academic achievers. A second group, "the spoilt", equally objected to eating the family meal but this group had different food prepared for them by their mothers. All but one of the group was male, most were the youngest child in the family, were white and working class, and many were either in employment or planned to leave education in the near future. For those not sharing the family meal, the outcome of negotiation within the family was, therefore, strongly influenced by gender. Among these was a third group of academically able young women who earned their independence and freedom from family constraint by catering for themselves. A fourth group are described as "the delegated", in that there was some sharing of responsibility within the family in determining both what should be eaten, and who should help in the preparation of meals. In this group, both young men and women shared in the cooking and this group was most likely to be in families in which both parents worked (Brannen et al. 1994).

The same study also illustrates how relationships within families changed once the young person entered the labour market. Relatively few young people had left education, and those who had were largely from white working-class backgrounds. For them, getting a job was often accompanied by being able to negotiate wider freedom about going out and the time at which they were expected to return. As is also reported by Jones, getting a job is also accompanied by the beginnings of a financial transaction between young people and their parents in which "board" money is paid (Jones 1991). This is not so much a means through which the cost of living at home is calculated and then met by the young person, as a symbolic act which is indicative of the way in which young workers are expected to start paying their way.

Brannen et al. also report on the problematic relationship between young people living with step-parents. None of the young men and only two young women picked their step-parent as the person with whom they got on best, although a small minority reported that they had excellent relationships with them. Young women, more so than young men, were more likely to report that they had "poor" or "very poor" relationships with a step-parent. This goes some way to explaining why, as both Kiernan and Jones report, they are more likely to leave the parental home at an early stage (Kiernan 1992, Jones 1994).

Families, households and leaving home

The research undertaken by Jones on the housing careers of young people suggested that it is useful to distinguish between households, families and homes (Jones 1993a). These distinctions can be made in the following terms and on the following grounds. Households usually refer to a number of adults and children who live together under one roof. They may or may not be involved in the sharing of resources, and in that sense negotiations within a household may be as complex as those we have described for families (Brannen et al. 1994). In families, the relationship between parent and child often involves the exercise of power and responsibilities and the granting of freedoms, all of which are constantly open to negotiation and renegotiation. Families are, therefore, the sites of both loving, caring and controlling relationships between members of a kinship group. The concept of "home", on the other hand, can be used to refer to both a territorial space, an identity, and a residential and emotional base. Jones has argued that young people regard "home" as "a secure, safe and private place of their own, and not dependent upon the presence of a family" (Jones 1993a: 5). So, even when a young person may be a member of a particular household or family, they may regard somewhere else as "home". Other young people, particularly where they are members of "reconstituted" families following a separation, divorce, bereavement or remarriage may feel they are members of more than one family, yet none of these may be properly regarded as "home". These distinctions are important in our discussion of the restructuring of family life in the past few decades. For while the bare facts of demography can tell us about household composition, they do little to illuminate what this means in terms of young people and family life, how these changes have created different notions of home, and how this in turn affects the transitions of youth. While these are areas which still need further conceptual exploration and empirical research, they are the beginnings of an important literature which can help to highlight the issues.

Until recently, little had been written about the early housing careers of young people (Ainley 1991, Furlong & Cooney 1990, Liddiard & Hutson 1991, Jones 1987, 1993a, 1993b, 1994). Jones, who has pioneered this area of research, suggests that we should not regard housing careers as linear in that young people may leave home and return on several occasions and for a variety of reasons. Sometimes the timing of leaving is a matter of choice and young people leave to enhance their educational or occupational career or to enter into a new partnership, living with someone else away from the parental home. Most moves away from the parental home are to allow young people to start a job or to continue their education, and most of these involve transitional housing of one sort or another (Jones 1993a). Moves are also temporary in that many students can move back to the family home during vacations and most have the option of returning home when their studies have been completed, or if they leave their job. The third "traditional" reason for leaving home, to set up a partnership or to get married, Jones reports as having declined in Scotland as elsewhere in Europe, and there are no reasons for thinking this does not apply to the rest of the United Kingdom (Jones 1993a).

Yet there are grounds to be concerned for young people who leave home for "negative" reasons, for, as Jones demonstrates, this is most likely to lead to negative consequences in terms of homelessness. In an analysis of a representative sample of young people who were aged 19 in 1991 and covered by the Scottish Young People's Survey (SYPS), 6% of those who had left home reported that they had been homeless since leaving. (SYPS is the Scottish equivalent of the Youth Cohort Study of England and Wales reported on in the last chapter.) Of these, six out of ten had left home because of family difficulties. A parallel study of young homeless Scots found the same proportion who had left home because of problematic relationships with parents, including more than a quarter of the homeless young people Jones studied who reported that they were "kicked out" (told to leave), and others who had left because of physical or sexual abuse (Jones 1993a). A third of those who had been homeless had been in care since the age of 14. A quarter had a step-parent and so family breakdown can be seen to have occurred at an early stage. (We will examine young people in and leaving care separately in Chapter 6.) Some young people leaving home early, including some who were told to leave by their parents, had precipitated the crisis by their own behaviour (drug taking, gambling and debt), and some were accepted back home at a later stage. Yet Jones does report correlations between the family circumstances in which they were living and their early home leaving.

Correlations are often complicated, with more than one feature in the background of young people contributing both to early leaving from the parental home and subsequent homelessness. Living in large families with more than two other brothers or sisters, having unemployment in the family, or young persons being unemployed themselves are all reported as associated with leaving home for negative, "non-traditional" reasons before the age of 19. Yet having a step-parent proved to be the main predictive correlate of leaving home, with nearly half of those living with a step-parent reporting having left home by the age of 19, compared to only 27% in intact families. Of these, nearly a quarter (23%) of young men, and four in ten young women gave family problems as their reason for leaving (Jones 1993a). This seems to confirm the other indications that young women are most restricted and controlled by the parents, that discipline from step-parents is often problematic and considered by young people to be illegitimate, and that young people's response to the difficulties they experience in stepfamilies is to leave home (often for negative reasons) much earlier than young people living in intact families (Brannen et al. 1994, Jones 1993a, 1994). Jones also examined the patterns of family support young people received from their parents as they left. Leaving home *per se* may be in the interests of both the young person and the family. Indeed, several of the young people interviewed by Jones and Gilliland reported that living alone had helped in the process of *feeling* more grown up (Jones & Gilliland 1993). Moves away from home still involve a negotiation of support from families, and it is to patterns of family support that we now turn.

Leaving home and family support

Jones examined patterns of family support for young people who left full-time education in Scotland at or near to minimum school-leaving age, and had left home for reasons other than to continue their education by an average age of around 19. This study is based on in-depth interviews with 26 young people from the Scottish Young People's Survey after they reached the age of 21 (Jones 1994). Half the group she studied had left home because of conflict with parents. Five of these were told to leave by their parents. The other half are grouped together according to three main types of reasons for leaving: forming new partnerships (4 cases); a desire for independence from the family (4 cases); moving away to get a job (5 cases). Nineteen of those who had initially left home returned home to live there again at some point before they were 21 years old, and fourteen were living there at the time of the interviews. This emphasizes the non-linear nature of housing careers. Ten young people had experienced homelessness in some form, and nine had children. The interviews examined the circumstances in which they had left and returned, and the financial, emotional and material support they had received from their families since initially leaving.

It should be remembered that when young people leave home, they are unlikely to receive much financial support from state benefits. In the last chapter we outlined a number of changes in social security arrangements which had weakened the support available for young people. Many of these covered the circumstances in which young people are eligible to receive benefit if they are not in full-time education, Youth Training or work. As we saw, this is only available in special circumstances to young people under the age of 18, and is paid at a specially reduced rate for 18–25-year-olds. In 1994, 16–17-year-olds receiving Income Support because they have been able to claim successfully that they are unable to live at home are entitled to £36.15 per week, slightly more than the rate granted in other circumstances. But since 1989, they have not been entitled to receive extra support to cover the cost of rent, rates or water rates. Since 1989, young people have been able to claim Housing Benefit, paid by local authorities rather than the Department of Social Security, and paid in arrears – something which does not help young people in immediate need. Housing Benefit is also difficult to claim, based upon what is assessed as a reasonable rent, and the evidence suggests that very few young people claim it (Davis 1994). Young people leaving home may, therefore, continue to be dependent upon their parents or others around them to provide them with the means of bare survival. Many live on very little income and starvation diets (Kirk et al. 1991).

In Jones's study of the main SYPS sample, financial support from parents was most likely to have been given where parents were in work and families intact. It was least likely to be given where young people had left stepfamilies or in lone-parent families which had financial difficulties of their own. Case studies of those followed up later indicated that, occasionally, step-parents had been supportive. Jones divided her sample into young people living in different family circumstances and examined the sort of support they received from their parents after they left home. Emotional support seems to be the least forthcoming from parents to young people leaving home early, but the emotional "climate" of support often improved over time. Many young people indicated that their families had given them material and financial assistance, often in the form of furniture, kitchen utensils and cooking equipment (Jones 1994). While half of those who left home had returned there again by the time of the study, some had incurred large debts. Many claimed to have learnt important lessons from their experiences and were determined to plan their next attempt to move away from home better. It is notable that it was the younger age group, aged 16 or 17, who received least support from their parents, and it is this group which is least eligible for the parsimonious financial support available from the state.

Youth transitions in the late 1990s
This chapter has reviewed how the circumstances in which young people grow up have been changed by transformations in family structure and patterns of family life. While the majority of young people are still brought up with both biological parents, as was outlined in the last chapter, more are economically dependent upon them for longer periods of time as extended transitions from school to work take them through ever longer periods of education and training. This chapter has further outlined that growing numbers of young people live in families which do not have two parents, and growing numbers experience the divorce or separation of their parents, and the reconstitution of families to involve step-parents. We have seen that these changes in family structure can affect family relationships and that these, in turn, can impact upon the main youth transitions. For most young people, their families are their major source of emotional, material and financial support as they attempt the precarious first steps towards adulthood. For a significant number of young people this support is far from secure, and in such circumstances they may experience unemployment, homelessness and destitution with little state support. In the remaining chapters of this book we will focus on particularly vulnerable young people. For these young people, growing up can be a frightening and unfulfilling experience which threatens their welfare and does little to enhance their involvement as full citizens of an adult society. Before turning to these vulnerable groups, however, we will examine what we mean by citizenship, how this has been influenced by social and economic trends, and how it has been revised by changes in the law.

Chapter Four

Youth citizenship and its changing context

Chapter 1 outlined a conceptualization of youth as a series of "transitions" from childhood to adulthood. The last two chapters further described the ways in which recent social and economic changes have restructured the status of "youth" in contemporary society and produced "extended" and "fractured" youth transitions. In describing these, and the processes through which the set of transitions seems to interrelate, particular attention has been drawn to the ways in which the welfares of different groups of young people have been affected. For some groups, "welfare" support can be argued to have declined over the past two decades and they have become significantly structurally disadvantaged in successfully making the transition to "adulthood" (Williamson 1993). In this sense, they have serious problems in being part of, and participating in, the community as full adult members. In the terms to be developed in this chapter, they are thus excluded from "citizenship". This chapter will examine what is meant by citizenship and how we can best conceptualize policies designed to enhance the citizenship of young people and ensure their welfare. It will also outline the changing policy context in which youth citizenship is to be understood. Chapter 5 considers the legal framework affecting young people's rights.

Citizenship and the welfare of young people

One of the major concepts developed to understand theoretically the advances made in Western societies in the development of welfare provision is that of "citizenship". T. H. Marshall argued, with particular reference to the development of the British welfare state at the end of the 1940s, that citizenship had evolved through three distinct phases covering three elements; civil, political and social citizenship (Marshall 1963). Each of the three elements he associated with a set of rights guaranteed for the individual by the state and made available through its institutions. The civil element is associated with individual freedoms and justice, "liberty of the person, freedom of speech, thought and faith, the right to own property and conclude valid contracts, and the rights to justice" (Marshall 1963: 74). The political element involves "rights to participate in the exercise of political power, as a member of a body invested with political authority or as an elector of the members of such a body" (p. 74). The social element refers to a wide range of entitlements from the right to be a recipient "of economic welfare and security [and] to the right to share to the full in the social heritage and to live the life of a civilised being according to the standards prevailing in the society" (p. 74). Marshall viewed these constellations of rights as being won through reforms spanning three centuries and culminating in the granting of social citizenship with the Beveridge and other welfare reforms at the end of the 1940s in the UK (Marshall 1963).

Despite writing at the beginning of the 1950s, Marshall's later writings showed that he was also aware of the complex ways in which rights were afforded to the various sectors of what he called a "hyphenated society" (Marshall 1981). This he saw as being made up not only of the individual and the state (including the welfare state) but also of industrial capitalism, the family and the voluntary sector. This is not the place to embark upon a critique of this notion of the "hyphenated society", but it must be emphasized that it is made up of a complex of legal frameworks and social institutions with different levels of authority, responsibility and duties. It is clear, furthermore, that this complex itself is subject to political manipulation and change, and has indeed altered considerably since the time when Marshall wrote.

Marshall recognized that the various sectors were potentially "at war" but in reality he regarded them as capable of compromise through which the rights to which he referred could be attained, considered legitimate, and enforced by a moral consensus. He assumed that this consensus could establish and regulate a social contract, not

CITIZENSHIP AND THE WELFARE OF YOUNG PEOPLE

just between the individual and the state but between industrial capitalism and the social institutions of its host society. Thus, individual citizens would not only be prepared to pay taxes to the state in return for benefits, but capitalists too would pay taxes to the state and offer work to its citizens in return for an educated, trained and motivated workforce. Furthermore, the state would both regulate the economy in the interests of full employment and provide the social infrastructure for the operation of capitalism.

While recognizing the importance of the three elements initially outlined by Marshall, Turner has argued that, most crucially, citizenship is concerned with the nature of the *social participation* of persons within the community (Turner 1990). Furthermore, he is more explicit than Marshall in noting that rights must be seen as part of a much wider social contract between the liberal state and capitalism. He also notes that "Citizenship is not simply about class and capitalism but also involves the social rights of women, children, the elderly and even animals." (Turner 1986) As we will see, the processes of inclusion, which grant citizenship to these groups, are problematic and several authors have suggested that, for these groups of people, citizenship is achieved "by proxy" being problematically based upon membership of a family unit with a (usually male) breadwinner (Jones & Wallace 1992, Lister 1991). But while much of the theoretical rhetoric of citizenship draws attention to the legal, social and economic processes and procedures of *inclusion*, we must also be equally concerned with, and aware of, the legal, social and economic processes of *exclusion*. Several authors have been critical of Marshall's notion of the evolutionary development of citizenship, arguing that the progress achieved in the 1940s could be, and arguably has been, just as easily put into reverse (Giddens 1982, Jessop 1988, Roche 1987, Turner 1990).

Marshall's initial essay on citizenship was based upon a number of theoretical and empirical assumptions which need to be challenged and revised. Indeed, the original conceptualization of citizenship can be seen as having been overtaken by events. A number of authors have pointed out that the society in which we now live is a fundamentally different economic, social and political world to the one in which Marshall developed his ideas (Roche 1992). As we saw in Chapters 2 and 3, some of our major social institutions, including the family, education and the labour market have been radically transformed. The nature of the economy and the operation of capitalism are also very different. Following a decade and a half of politics and social policy making dominated by the right of the political spectrum, it is simply not good enough naïvely to apply an unrevised concept. This is because it was originally based upon a notion of welfare ushered in by a reforming Labour government operating within completely different social and economic conditions. In seeking to develop and apply the concept of citizenship to an understanding of the rights of young people, we must begin with a thorough and far-reaching re-examination of both the meaning of the term and of the new conditions and contexts in which it is to be applied. This chapter will provide an appraisal of a series of basic theoretical and empirical assumptions upon which Marshall's schema can be seen to rest.

Citizenship and different categories of citizen

First, it is clear that Marshall did not fully explore the ways in which different status groups in society were granted different kinds of citizenship. He regarded "the adult male [as] the citizen *par excellence*" (Marshall 1963: 84) but this, of course, leaves problematic the status of the bulk of the population who are neither male nor adult. Feminist writers, from the eighteenth century onwards, have made claims to aspects of citizenship for women, but have often done so while asserting that they wanted to be equal *but different* (Walby 1994). Furthermore, although some of the rights they wished to claim could be held to be those of universal citizenship (to vote, to hold property in their own name, for instance), many others are rights which may be regarded as being of particular importance to women as a distinct group (rights to abortion, rights to protection against rape within marriage, rights against sexual harassment at work, rights to child care for women workers, etc.). Citizenship must, therefore, not only be capable of specifying universal rights but must also be capable of addressing the sectional rights of different categories of citizen who live in different social, economic and material conditions. Our task in this chapter is to begin to identify the distinctive rights which may be claimed by young people.

Rights and duties

Writers from a variety of different political perspectives have called attention to the fact that, in developing his theory of citizenship, Marshall concentrates upon the winning of rights but pays little attention to the duties which are attendant upon them (Mann 1987, Murray 1984, Plant 1988, Roche 1992). Yet, the two sides of the equation are inextricably linked. If someone can be said to have rights, then these must be rights *over* some other person, group of people, or social institution. It should be recognized immediately that this statement implies that rights can involve claims against both individuals and public and private bodies, including (but certainly not exclusively confined to) publicly accountable agencies of the state. If we can be said to have rights, then some body (or somebody) must have corresponding duties towards us. And if rights are to mean anything, these public and private bodies must have the obligation, ability and resources to fulfil them. At its simplest, if I have a right to be told the truth, then someone else has the obligation to be honest. If I have the right to knowledge about something, then someone else must be identified as having the duty and responsibility to provide that knowledge and the means and ability of doing so. If I have the right to some form of housing or social care, then somebody or some body must be identified as responsible for providing it. Without such a clear specification of responsibilities and obligations which mirror rights, the rhetoric concerning them lacks real substance, becoming a slogan in search of an enemy, or vacuous, in-principle policy statements, without the practical means of implementation.

While this knitting together of rights and responsibilities may, at first sight, be regarded as merely a means of giving the concept of rights a more directed policy agenda, it should also be recognized that their tying together has most vociferously been advocated and defended by critics of welfare provision from the New Right (Gilder 1982, Major 1993, Mead 1986, Murray 1984, Novak 1987). A number of influential authors have argued that in order to qualify for welfare, and as a condition of welfare being given, citizens should first be expected to fulfil the duties and responsibilities society can reasonably expect of them (Major 1993, Mead 1986, Murray 1990). So, for instance, a right to education is mirrored by a duty to learn; a right to work is matched by a duty to earn; and the right to receive welfare support from the state must be met by a duty to contribute, in some way, to the community which gives it.

Contingencies and balance of rights and duties

At its most simple, claims about rights and duties are made within particular sectors of welfare. So, for instance, for some critics of welfare, the right to social security benefit when a person is unemployed, must be tied to a willingness to work (and accept any job which is available), and/or a willingness to be re-trained so as to be employable in a labour market with shifting skill needs. This limitation specifying a conditional or contingent notion of entitlement to welfare while unemployed is what is meant by "workfare" (Walker 1991). There are some authors who have argued that participation in the labour market is *the* key to all other rights, and that other rights (such as access to child care) should be developed in order for this paramount right to be fulfilled (Lister 1990). But there are dangers in such a position. Rights to maternity leave and child support are closely related to the rights and needs of children, as much as to the rights (or obligation) of women to participate in the labour market. Some writers from the Right of the political spectrum have argued that, in considering the rights and obligations of women as mothers, we must balance their obligations to their children with any expectation that they should engage in paid employment (Gilder 1986). Indeed, some have gone so far as to suggest a system of "learnfare" rather than "workfare", through which women's obligation to "participate" in the community can be gauged by the satisfactory attendance of their children at school (see discussion by Roche 1992).

This is not the place to enter into this wide-ranging debate. But it is clear that rights and obligations involve a complex set of relationships which span public and private institutions. Within the family especially, balancing the rights and obligations of the different parties is extremely complex. Children, it is claimed by some, may have rights of privacy, rights of association, and rights to free recreation (Franklin 1986, Freeman 1983). Yet parents have responsibilities for supervision, and responsibilities for the care and control of "children". In some circumstances these rights and responsibilities are potentially in conflict. If children use "privacy" in a way that threatens their welfare (through drug abuse for instance), then parents have a duty to intervene. If children use their rights of association and recreation to create welfare harm for others in the community (through truanting, vandalism, crime, or associating with people who might encourage such "anti-social" activity), then do parents not have a duty to intervene? Certainly, family welfare policy suggests that they have. For, where parents do not exercise proper care and control of their children, the state (through the powers of the courts) may intervene and legally replace the responsibilities of biological parenthood with legal guardianship of its own. Balancing the rights and responsibilities of adults, children and young people across public and private institutions is therefore an immensely complex matter.

Part of this complexity is caused by the fact that parents can be held responsible to public institutions for the behaviour of their children and the care and control they exercise over them. And where parental care and control breaks down to such an extent that the welfare needs of children (and young people) are threatened, public institutions and public servants (such as the courts and social workers) have a right and a duty to intervene, *in the best interests of the child*. This balancing of the rights and responsibilities both within the family, and between the family and the state, will be examined further when we discuss changes in the legal context of "citizenship" in the next chapter. For the issues which have been addressed in this section were very much the focus of the debates which led to both The Children Act 1989 and The Criminal Justice Act 1991. Before turning to the legal context of citizenship, further theoretical clarifications need to be made.

Rights, needs, interests and access to resources

Within the arena of family policy, especially, there is a recognizable tension in the balancing of needs, rights and interests (Parton 1991). We must, therefore, be clear about what these concepts mean, and how they relate to the rationale and administration of welfare for young people. *Rights*, as we have seen, are part of the *political rhetoric of citizenship*. Within this, as Franklin among others has pointed out, two kinds of rights can be identified: *legal rights* or entitlements and *moral rights* which may not be a legal entitlement but may be a desirable end to be achieved by future legislation and welfare development

(Franklin 1986). Furthermore, as Barbalet and others have indicated, in order to have any meaning rights must be connected to the *abilities and resources* of people to fulfil those rights (Barbalet 1988). Without such a commitment to develop abilities and commit resources, moral "rights" become little more than a social policy "wish list".

Needs too have been argued to be at the heart of social policy analysis and policy making and to constitute a *social policy rhetoric* of welfare analysis. In a wide-ranging and thorough exploration of the concept, Doyal & Gough argue that what makes social needs distinct is first, that they may be claimed to be universal and secondly, that "if individual needs are not satisfied . . ., then serious harm of some specified and objective kind will result" (Doyal & Gough 1992). For Doyal & Gough, needs analysis, therefore, must attempt to be objective and not political or normative (in the sense of being based upon subjective judgement). As a result, social policy is able to aid the development of welfare services designed according to measured need. They further argue that the most basic needs include not only *material needs* (survival or health needs) but what they term *autonomy and learning needs*, through which individuals are given both a sufficient sense of their own identity and the skills, knowledge and freedoms to act as autonomous individuals. To meet both material needs and autonomy and learning needs, they argue, requires the allocation of resources. Although Doyal & Gough discuss needs in general, some of those they identify can be seen to be of fundamental importance to young people. Other authors, rather than arguing that needs are necessarily universal and applicable to all people equally, have suggested that it is important also to focus on the different needs of different categories of people (Baldwin & Hirst 1994, Barnes 1991, Glendinning & Millar 1987). In this sense children, young persons, mothers, and the retired can be said to have different needs. Campbell, for instance, has argued that "each person ought to receive or be left in possession of that which is necessary to meet his or her basic course-of-life need" (Campbell 1983: 134).

A third concept which is sometimes used interchangeably with rights and needs is that of *interests*. But interests are more clearly sectional and illustrate a potential or actual conflict between claims to rights made by sectional groups. So, for instance, within a family, the interests of the child may be in conflict with the interests of parents. In adjudicating the balance of rights, responsibilities and duties between public institutions, similar sectional disputes can be seen to occur. As was argued in Chapter 2, for example, in the framing of education policy, the interests of industry in developing particular vocational skills may be in conflict with the interests of liberal educationalists, who, like Marshall, may wish to defend the right of the child to "share to the full in the social heritage . . . [of] society". At another very basic level, the interests of welfare claimants may be seen to be in conflict with the interests of tax payers. Often the rhetoric of needs and interests may be confusingly used interchangeably, most notably when policy is recommended which claims that the *interest* of the child must be paramount, as a means of fulfilling its *needs*. But here it is important to recognize that the best *interests of the child* are being argued for on the basis of its *needs*, i.e. related to the potential for serious and significant welfare harm through not providing for these *needs*.

Children and young people's rights

Franklin has argued for a specific set of rights for children (Franklin 1986: 14). He suggests these can be classified into four main types: welfare rights, protection rights, adult rights, rights against parents. The first of these, welfare rights, include rights to nutrition, medical services, housing and education. Protective rights are designed to protect the child against inadequate care, neglect or physical or emotional abuse. The argument for adult rights suggests that young people are excluded from these (the rights to vote, work, marry and drive, for instance) by what Franklin and others regard as arbitrary and irrational chronological age criteria. Freeman has similarly argued that the arbitrary nature of age-related rights could and should be replaced by criteria which are based more upon the capacity of young people to display properly the skills and duties involved in exercising these rights (Freeman 1983). Franklin's final category, "children rights", suggests too that, rather than having all autonomy in decision making denied until some arbitrary age(s) of majority, these rights should be granted earlier, though again this should be conditional upon the capacity of young people to exercise their responsibilities properly. The issues of autonomy he details in this category range from choice about length of hair and what a young person should eat, to decisions about recreation, leaving home, and independence in decisions about health care, including contraception and abortion. Franklin seems to regard his last category as largely concerned with rights against parents, but given his examples it is clear it might also include rights against social institutions, such as schools, institutions of residential care and medical practices.

Franklin's discussion highlights several issues of importance in discussing rights. First, rights are concerned with emancipation; allowing people to make and exercise their own choices. But protection rights and welfare rights also involve curtailing freedoms. This is often argued on the grounds of acting in a child's best *interests* or, more accurately, making certain that its needs are adequately met. So, for instance, prohibiting young people from engaging in paid work, or restricting the kinds of work they do or the hours and conditions in which they can work, can all be argued for on the grounds of health, safety or a paramount need that they should spend appropriate amounts of time and effort on their education. Secondly, it is important to recognize that in diminishing young people's freedoms because of some paramount *need or interest*, there is conflict between whose interest is being served. In some circumstances, as for instance in the case of abuse, this might involve separating a child from its family to protect it from serious harm (i.e. that dealing with the child's *needs* is paramount and should in some cases overrule any rights parents might have in the care and control of their children). In other cases, in for instance requiring a child or young person to undertake compulsory education, the balancing of *interests* involved seems to be more complex.

Marshall himself argues for the importance of education as a social welfare right of young people as the fulfilment of an adult right to be educated (Marshall 1963). Yet he is also clear that "when the state guarantees that all children should be educated . . . the aim of education is to *shape* the future adult" (p. 84, emphasis added). As will be seen when changes in the education system itself are examined, this "shaping" is not altogether done in the interests of the citizen as an individual (whether child or adult), but with the needs and interests of labour market and the wider community in mind. The third issue of importance in Franklin's discussion is the awkwardness with which he conflates children and young people. To be fair, in his discussion of the arbitrary nature of age-related rights, he does recognize that the rights to be accorded to 3-year-olds can, quite reasonably, be different from those granted to those aged 16 or 20. Furthermore, he and others (including those responsible for framing the Children Act 1989), have argued that the capacities of a set of young people of the same chronological age might differ enormously and, accordingly, that the awarding of rights should be related to the capability of the young person to exercise them properly and responsibly (Freeman 1983, Parton 1991). This, of course, begs lots of questions as to how this can be assessed.

A distinctive youth perspective on citizenship

From the point of view of this book, it is inadequate to conflate childhood and youth. For, as was argued in Chapter 1, while childhood and adulthood can be distinguished in terms of dependency and independency, youth can be regarded as a state of relative *semi-independency* and autonomy during which young people go through a series of "staged progressions" to the independency of the adult. This is in line with the conceptualization of youth as a series of transition processes, which was introduced in Chapter 1. Given this, in focusing on young people's rights, needs, and interests it is necessary to identify a distinct set of rights which clearly relate to specific aspects of each of these transitions and how they interrelate.

In their important discussion of youth and citizenship, Jones & Wallace make a number of very useful points (Jones & Wallace 1992). First, they argue that, in examining young people's rights we must examine what they call both the "public" and "private" spheres and the ways in which these interrelate. In particular, they rightly suggest that we must open "the black box" of family relationships (the private sphere) and examine how these relationships within the family interface with the roles and relationships young people have with social institutions external to the family (Jones & Wallace 1992). Chapter 3 of this book attempted to demonstrate and illustrate the importance of this by reviewing the limited research evidence about family relationships and young people. Secondly, Jones & Wallace agree that we should concentrate our attention on the processes of youth transitions, rather than on arbitrary chronological age ranges. Thirdly, they remind us of the interlocking nature of young people's rights and that access to one set of rights seems to be dependent upon access to others. This, they argue, makes it crucial that we fully examine "the maze of public and private institutions structuring . . . youth" (p. 142), and call for "a more holistic approach to young people's needs" (p 155). This is made clearer by a fourth important argument.

Jones & Wallace argue that the balance between freedoms, rights and parental control within the family are inextricably linked to the economic dependency young people have on their parents. Following Barbalet, they further argue that in establishing rights, we must be concerned not only with legal entitlements but with the ability of individuals to mobilize resources to fulfil such entitlements (Barbalet 1988). Taking both these points together, what follows is that we must recognize that the ability to "mobilize resources" can be based, not on some legal universal entitlement (to education, for instance), but upon access to private resources which, for young people, is through parents. These resources are, of course, far from evenly distributed. Young people's ability to exercise what may be a legal right is, therefore, undermined by the economic inequalities of the parents' generation and especially their differential ability financially to support their children during an extended period of economic dependency. Without the commitment of sufficient resources to match rights, a universal legal entitlement for young people can be undermined by the lack of availability of resources through parental financial support.

Yet, although it is possible to agree broadly with all of these points, and while they may aid the development of a notion of youth citizenship, they certainly do not add up to a clear catalogue of young people's rights. They raise important questions and issues for the conceptualization of youth citizenship without providing definitive answers in terms of young people's rights. Furthermore, Jones & Wallace, despite arguing that we should concentrate upon the transition processes and develop a holistic approach (aimed at a better understanding of how the elements of the different transition processes interrelate), set great store on the critical importance of only one of them – economic independence (mainly through paid employment) – as *the* key which unlocks access to a whole range of other rights. Following Lister's analysis of women and citizenship, they argue that full citizenship for young people is possible only where there is economic independence (Lister 1990, 1991). Otherwise young people only attain "citizenship by proxy" in which their rights are considerably eroded by economic dependence on family breadwinners, and any universality of transition rights is undermined by an increasing likelihood of longer periods of dependency upon the parent generation.

While not wishing to deny the importance of economic independence, there are potential dangers in focusing too much attention on this as *the only* key to youth citizenship. It may, indeed, be particularly important for the ability to exercise consumer citizenship (access to choice in what and how we consume) which Jones & Wallace also consider to be important. Yet, to focus too much upon one element of the transition process is to deflect attention from rights, entitlements, the availability of opportunities, and access to resources in others. And to focus too much on the benefits which might accrue from the fulfilment of *a right to work* may deflect from *rights at work* and rights in other spheres such as autonomy and knowledge rights in education and training, or the rights of young people in care. It is for this reason that it is important to focus on the rights which pertain to *all* the transition processes outlined in Chapter 1, and, as will be shown, it is these which constitute the distinctiveness of *young people's rights*. If a set of transition needs and transition rights can be clearly established, then this will enable the evaluation of youth policy according to whether it meets the specific and distinctive needs of young people in successfully making these transitions. Furthermore, if these rights and needs can be identified, then they can be used in the evaluation of welfare policies and practices, according to whether these either enhance or diminish the welfares of young people in making the transitions to the full citizenship of adulthood.

Before concluding this section, the relationship between needs, rights, and interests and how this relates to access to resources should be made clear. An assessment of needs, it has been argued, provides a basis for social policies. The prevention of serious welfare harm is the first call citizens can make upon social welfare and can, as Marshall argued, constitute social rights. Following Doyal & Gough, serious welfare harm can be argued to result not only from failure to provide for basic material survival, but also if the conditions and resources for individual autonomy are not fostered and developed. In this sense, meeting needs is not merely a process of paternalistic welfare administration, but a process of liberation and empowerment.

Rights involve both legally and enforceable claims on others in both private and public institutions, and rights to resources. We must be careful not to restrict the listing of rights to a catalogue of *existing* laws. To be of more use in setting a policy agenda, a Charter of Rights must be a manifesto for political reform and change, and rights must be properly regarded as making moral, as well as legal, claims. A social policy agenda for youth will, therefore, include a generic claim that young people should be accorded the right to have their basic needs fulfilled. But a social policy agenda must do more than that, for it can provide a more developed programme for the reform of specific institutions targeted at the incremental improvement of the welfare of young people undertaking the transitions to adulthood. The point can be illustrated with one example concerning young people being brought up in the public care (in children's homes or in foster care). As we will argue in Chapter 6, such young people should not suffer additional disadvantages in education, training, or the access to employment opportunities as a result of being brought up in care. Their needs (defined in terms of the avoidance of welfare harm) should be paramount in drawing up the aims and objectives of care systems, and young people's rights (including the right not to be disadvantaged) built into the design and management of care regimes. A social policy of young people in care must be based upon a critical evaluation of the impact of being brought up in care on the main youth transition processes and provide more specific programmes of reform designed to protect young people's rights and better meet their needs. A similar point could be made for other groups of young people, such as those with disabilities and special needs, to be discussed in Chapter 7. This interface between needs, rights and how they can be used to develop more specific social policy agendas is, therefore, the basis of subsequent chapters of this book.

Before we turn to these special cases, it is also important to recognize in general terms that the context within which needs are identified and rights developed is one that involves many different and competing interests. Rights involve claims against others. The meeting of needs often requires making resources available which must be released by others. Social policy making requires both the balancing of different interests and the making of claims on resources. All this takes place within a political domain. As we will see in the next chapter, legal rights can be, and have been, taken away as well as given, and so the social policy agenda is both a moral, legal and political battlefield. It is for this reason that, in developing a social policy for youth which is designed to enhance citizenship, we must be keenly aware of the contemporary legal and moral contexts of policy debates. Fraser has argued that "this peculiar juxtaposition of a discourse about needs with discourses about rights and interests is one of the distinctive marks of late-capitalist political culture" (Fraser 1984). Marshall too was very much aware that legal rights are not the only means through which citizenship is granted. Of particular importance is the provision of welfare through the operation of private and public, social and economic institutions. The social, political and economic world has been subject to much radical change since Marshall's initial essay. It is to this changing empirical and policy context of citizenship that we now turn.

The changing social, economic and political context

In his attempt to review and rethink the meaning of citizenship for the contemporary world, Maurice Roche has argued that a number of major trends must be taken on board (Roche 1992). In Chapters 2 and 3 we reviewed some of the major ways in which youth transitions have been transformed by social and economic changes taking place during the last quarter of the twentieth century. Sociological literature has been awash with attempts to depict the nature of the new epoch in theoretical terms (Bauman 1992, Burrows & Loader 1994, Harvey 1989, Lash 1990, Smart 1993). It has been described as both "post" and "ized": post-industrial, post-fordist, post-modern, post-national; globalized, localized, individualized, and even McDonaldized (Featherstone 1990, Ritzer 1993, Robertson 1990). It is not necessary to enter into the debates surrounding the attempt to depict these conditions, but it is important to recognize some of the institutional shifts to which these theories elude, and the social policy debates which have surrounded them. For, as Roche points out, they do substantially effect the ways in which it is possible to rethink the meaning of citizenship (Roche 1992). In briefly outlining this changing context for our understanding of citizenship, the focus will be on a number of important institutional areas affecting young people and the major shifts in the policy agenda which have occurred in recent years.

The challenge to the assumption of full employment

In proclaiming the triumphs of citizenship in Britain, Marshall was writing in the wake of the Beverage welfare reforms designed, in part, to attack the dis-welfares of unemployment, and in an era which accepted Keynesian economic management as one of the principal weapons of the state. At the time he was writing, maintaining "full employment" was assumed to be one of the main duties of government and one which it was largely possible to fulfil. But the assumption that the industrial capitalist economy could maintain full employment has been rudely challenged by the persistently high rates of unemployment since the 1970s and widespread and long-term unemployment in the 1980s and 1990s. Furthermore, this unemployment has been argued to be structural rather than cyclical and, as such, not so much precipitated by temporary swings in the trade cycle, as linked to permanent and irreversible changes in the capitalist system itself. In particular, the description of widespread structural unemployment is supported by evidence of collapse in the wealth-creating manufacturing sector of the economy. Patterns of growth in the labour market during periods of economic recovery have taken the form of an increased number of jobs in the service sector, rather than a recovery of employment prospects in manufacturing. Both American and British authors have claimed that this signals a change from an industrial to a post-industrial society (Bell 1974, Standing 1986). This change has meant a fundamental transformation of the demand side of the labour market – a switch of labour demand from manufacturing to service industries. During the 1970s and 1980s some industries, such as coal, steel and shipbuilding, collapsed and contracted. Others such as textiles relocated to the Third World. Still more became increasingly dependent upon technology and switched their labour demands accordingly. These economic changes have left whole zones of industry abandoned (the growth of the "rust belt"). Whole cities and regions are blighted with structural and long-term unemployment, leading to the growth of destitute communities encamped alongside derelict factories and with little chance of local economic regeneration capable of mopping up the high levels of local unemployment created by structural change.

As was pointed out in Chapter 2, the British government's policy response to unemployment has been somewhat limited by both its commitment to curbing public expenditure, and a belief that it was only from private employers and private enterprise that any sustainable upturn in labour demand would come. Until recently, policy makers from across the political spectrum have resisted the assumption that we can return to "full employment" (Commission on Social Justice 1994, McLaughlin 1994). As was argued in Chapter 2, changes in labour market policy have eroded young people's rights to, and at, work. Restrictions on the working hours of young people have been abandoned, as have restrictions on the conditions in which they work.

Changes in family patterns

Changes in family structure and family relationships were reviewed in Chapter 3. It is noteworthy, however, that Marshall's concept of citizenship was based upon an unexplored assumption about the stability of family life which is difficult to sustain in the 1990s. The development of the British welfare state, and Marshall's description of it, both made fundamental assumptions about the ways in which the family provided welfare for its members (Marshall 1963). While Beveridge and other writers were explicit in their recognition of the role of the private and voluntary sectors in continuing to help in delivering some aspects of welfare (such as private insurance and private education), the largest voluntary and private provider of welfare (the family) was largely taken for granted. Workers (and breadwinners) were assumed to be male and adult. Women as unpaid housewives and mothers supported by male breadwinners were assumed to be the norm. Women were, it is true, granted special welfare provisions, but these were largely confined to benefits for marriage, separation or widowhood, rights to a pension and allowances for their children. Their contribution to the funding of the welfare state through National Insurance was also different from male earners, again because the assumption was that the majority would continue to contribute indirectly through their life-long husbands. The benefit system was thus rigidly sex segregated and based upon the assumption of the traditional, life long, nuclear family.

Young people too were assumed for the most part to be unproblematically integrated into the civilization of nuclear families. These would socialize them into appropriate lifestyles and aspirations, ensure their participation in appropriate education and training, steer them clear of crime and anti-social behaviour, and care for them and protect them until such time as they emerged from the chrysalis of family life to be full-fledged adults. Properly functioning families with male breadwinners and women carers were taken for granted, as was the fulfilment of parental duties in the provision of primary care and day-to-day control of their children. As we saw in Chapter 3, both these assumptions are hugely challenged by developments in family structure over the past two decades.

In the United States, an expansion of the number of divorces and single-parent families led to the New Right's concern with an "underclass", which Murray among others sees as also threatening to appear in Britain (Murray 1990, Smith 1992). At its most crude and strident, the New Right's concern with the underclass is not so much to do with the creation of groups of citizens divorced from civil, political and social rights, as with the growth of a self-perpetuating culture permanently detached from the responsibilities of work, and mother-and-father dual parenting, and surviving at the expense of others in the community, by feeding their drug-dependency with the proceeds of crime. Given this list, it is of little wonder that the moral panic about the underclass has been seen as a moral vilification of "idle, thieving bastards" (Bagguley & Mann 1992). There is some variation of position among New Right writers. Some, such as Lawrence Mead, argue that the evidence shows that at least half of all American single mothers seek work and are in employment, but despite this they remain part of the "working poor" (Mead 1986). Others, such as George Gilder and Charles Murray, regard workfare arrangements for women with children to be a disaster, arguing that "female domination of work among the poor is the problem, not the solution" and will "only accelerate family decay". For both Gilder and Murray, women's place is in the home and their contribution to the state should be seen as adequately bringing up children and in particular "taming teenage boys" (as quoted in Roche 1992).

In Britain, the policy responses to these issues have been largely confined to attempts to encourage parental authority within the family (through the Criminal Justice Acts 1991 and 1994), and parental financial responsibility (through the Child Support Act 1992), although there have been verbal attacks on the welfare entitlements of single mothers (in particular around the Conservative Party Conference in 1993). So far, Britain has resisted the temptation formally to implement "workfare" or "learnfare" policies for single mothers, although one of the themes of the Conservative Party Conference in 1993 was the return to traditional family values, with more than one speech indicating that single mothers could not expect preferential treatment (in housing for instance) from the welfare state. For the moment, family policy in Britain is directed towards encouraging family responsibility rather than penalizing single parents. But the existence of life-long two-parent families supporting young people and providing for their welfare no longer constitutes an empirical assumption that can be made. This has considerable importance for claims for state support for young people who are attempting the transitions of youth.

The European context to rights
In both employment and family policy there have been significant developments, but ones which do not suggest an enhancement of the welfare careers of most groups of young people. Yet there is another, more optimistic, arena. The British government makes repeated claims that unemployment is an international problem, a European problem and one determined by the global economy. Much of the funding for positive unemployment and training measures, and regional development aid, has come from the European Community (now Union), with regional policy and training measures heavily subsidized from the European Social Fund. In framing a positive agenda for rights, it is, therefore, important to examine this wider European dimension. It is of some significance that much of the underwriting of rights to and at work is made by European institutions, and many of the resources allocated to the fulfilment of these rights are provided by European funds.

Comparatively little has been written about young people's rights as laid down through European institutions. Given this, and the importance such rights have for the welfare of young people in the next century, their main scope and potential will be outlined. The legal basis of the European Economic Community was the Treaty of Rome 1957. This contained vague references to "the harmonization of social systems", and a more specific shopping list of social policy issues through article 117, to a "close co-operation in matters such as employment, labour law and working conditions, vocational training, social security and health and safety at work". This policy agenda remained largely dormant until the 1980s, and until the late 1980s it seemed more of a "wish list" than something which could be developed into a meaningful charter of social rights. In 1986 the Treaty of Rome was amended by the Single European Act and a number of authors have drawn attention to the potential of the European Social Charter (ESC) it embraced (Brewster & Teague 1989, Coote 1992).

Part 1 of the ESC lists 19 rights which include: the right to protection of health (article 11); the right to social security (article 12); the right to social and medical assistance (article 13); the right to benefit from social welfare services (article 14); the right of the family to social welfare services (article 16); and the right of mothers and children to social and economic protection (article 17). Other articles within the Charter refer to rights which are specifically directed to the needs of young people and other groups with special needs. These include the right to vocational guidance, the right to vocational training, and the right of those with physical or mental disabilities to vocational training rehabilitation and social resettlement. A further Protocol to the ESC was adopted in 1988. This covers: the right to equal opportunities and equal treatment in matters of employment and occupation without discrimination on the grounds of sex (article 1); the right to information and consultation at the workplace (article 2); the right to take part in the determination and improvement of working conditions and the working environment (article 3); the right of elderly persons to social protection, to the provision of adequate resources, to housing adapted to their needs, and the rights of those in institutional care (article 4). In May 1989, the European Commission produced a Community Charter of Fundamental Social Rights for Workers.

Many of these developments have been hotly disputed by the British government. At the Madrid Summit in June 1989, there was considerable resistance to further European intervention in social policy areas. Since the Madrid summit, there has been much insistence by the British government, in particular, on the *principle of subsidiarity*: that issues should only be decided at a Community level where the same broad policy objectives cannot be achieved by actions of individual sovereign states. At Strasburg, in December 1989, Britain indicated that it would refuse to sign the new Social Charter and at Maastricht Britain insisted on a "Social Protocol", through which it opted out of the social policy agenda as laid down in the "Social Chapter" of the Maastricht Treaty. Despite the "Social Chapter" being a major political issue for the Conservative Party, both the main opposition parties in Britain remain committed to its implementation. Yet, in all the heated political debate about the Maastricht Treaty, there was a strange silence about the fact that the government remained committed to many aspects of the Social Action Programme; the means through which the Social Chapter will be implemented. Furthermore, it expects to be able to sign up to most of the proposals (Employment Department 1992).

The Maastricht Treaty 1992, which came into force in November 1993, was the latest of a series of moves towards the economic, political and social union of European countries. A single market (introduced in 1993) is regarded by most European countries as much more than a means of bringing down import and export regulations and tariffs. Rather, it is regarded as being a move towards the development of "a level playing field" for the production and marketing of goods. This involves a harmonization of conditions of work and the entitlements of workers. The European Social Charter and the "Social Chapter" of the Maastricht Treaty are, therefore, potentially very important in the development of young people's rights.

Britain, under the Major Government has argued that *some elements* of the Social Chapter of Maastricht involve unnecessary and damaging interference in employer–employee relations and will ultimately cost jobs. But it has continued to take part in intergovernmental conferences on employment, skill training, health and safety, equal opportunities, and the needs of people with disabilities. There is still debate as to how the Social Chapter of the Maastricht Treaty will be implemented. European policy can take three distinct forms: "directives", "regulations", and "opinions and advice". The most likely form of social policy intervention affecting young people is through EC "directives" which bind member states to policy "objectives", but leave it up to nation states as to the form and methods through which the objectives are achieved. Failure to implement directives can, however, be challenged in the European courts.

In some areas of the Maastricht agreement, the British government is currently insisting on exemption from European directives. In the Directive on Young People and Employment, negotiated in October 1993, Britain claimed a six-year (renewable) "opt-out" from restrictions placed on the employment of young people, and threatened to fight any moves to insist on its implementation in Britain in the European courts. The government has argued that

> The UK fully supports the need to safeguard the health and safety of *all* workers, and recognises that young people may need extra protection given their relative immaturity. However, specific restrictions on the work of young people above the minimum school leaving age are only justified where the health and safety hazards are greater than for adults. Additionally, there is a widespread agreement amongst employers and other interested bodies that it is essential not to price young workers out of the labour market. Imposition of regulations that add to the business costs in respect of young workers will deter employers from recruiting new entrants to the labour market. (Employment Department 1992: 21)

As regards the Directive on Vocational Training, however, Britain seems happy to accept implementation. In June 1992, the EEC adopted the directive which gives every community national certain rights to have qualifications gained in one member state recognized or taken into account in other member states where entry to a job is regulated on the basis of specific national qualifications. The Maastricht Treaty respects the diversity of individual countries' training systems, but under the EC directive, Britain's system of National Vocational Qualifications (NVQs) has been recognized throughout Europe for the first time. Britain has also accepted much of European policy on specific aid programmes for people with disabilities.

It is not within the scope of this chapter to adjudicate the rights and wrongs of this "pick and choose" approach to European Social Policy. Nor should it indulge in crystal ball gazing as to whether the broad thrust of the Maastricht agreements on social policy will be a temporary blip of European interference in British sovereignty or the beginning of a new chapter in pan-national social rights. What is clear is that there *is* a European context to policy development, and that this is underwritten by a European Social Fund which funds policy implementations. It is therefore of vital importance that we should recognize this European dimension of social policy in considering youth policy and youth rights as an agenda for change in the twenty-first century.

Chapter Five

Youth and citizenship: the legal context of young people's rights

The last chapter introduced the concept of citizenship and discussed how it helped our understanding of the rights, needs and interests of young people. It was argued that what made young people's rights, needs and interests distinctive was a concern for the main youth transitions described in Chapter 1. A social policy agenda informed by this approach is concerned, therefore, with the creation of a welfare environment in which young people can, at an appropriate point in their life, move from education to the labour market, be less dependent upon their families, and live independently of them. It was further argued in the last chapter that it was useful to distinguish between needs, rights and interests. The identification of needs involves establishing conditions under which serious welfare harm will result should needs not be met. So, for instance, it can be claimed that young people need to be brought up under conditions which will minimize their risk of being unemployed, socially isolated or homeless – the serious welfare harm which results from failed youth transitions. Furthermore, meeting such needs implies not merely ensuring that young people live in appropriate social, material and emotional circumstances, but fostering and developing their ability to make informed and wise decisions about their future career development. In this sense, young people have a need for their autonomy to be enhanced as they approach the transitions of youth.

Claiming rights, on the other hand, involves making legal or moral claims on public or private bodies. Many of the rights claimed for children, following Marshall, can be seen to be social rights in the sense of being demands that proper levels of welfare are delivered by the institutions on which children are dependent (Marshall 1963). Children's rights involve claims that they should have their needs met, that they should be protected from abuse and neglect, and that they should not suffer welfare harm. Rights involving adults and young people, on the other hand, also involve claims to freedoms, autonomy and responsibilities of action and decision making, and as such are, in Marshall's terms, political and civil rights. In that many rights of children, adults and young people involve claims against others, rights often involve the balancing of the legitimate interests of different parties in any potential dispute. Interests thus refer to the claims made by different sections of society, or different parties within an institution. So, for instance, children's rights are often expected to be fulfilled within families by their parents, or by agencies of the welfare state such as the health and education services. And in fulfilling these rights, there are potential conflicts of interest. Within the family there are, on occasions, differences between the interests of children, parents and the wider community in determining by whom, and how, social control should be exercised. In discussing education provision in Chapter 2 we also reviewed the debates concerning the content and accountability of education. So, as we saw, industrialists, parents, teachers and young people all have different claims on the provision of education, but from differing perspectives. Politicians have attempted to adjudicate between these different interests in different ways at different points in time.

The balancing of needs, rights and interests is, therefore, very much a political act and one in which the law and the interpretation and implementation of the law is of considerable importance. The law is an important means through which rights are established and through which duties and responsibilities are defined. The last chapter examined the social and economic context in which young people's welfare must be understood. In this chapter we examine the ways in which the law has been revised to meet the changing circumstances in which young people grow up. It is, of course, impossible in one short chapter to outline every detail of the laws affecting young people, or even to catalogue all the ways in which their legal entitlements have changed in recent years. But it is important to detail some of the major political debates and changes in the law which have taken place within the last decade, for these help us to understand some of the theoretical and empirical issues raised in the last chapter. As we will see, the law has much to say about the rights and responsibilities of young people, and how, and under what circumstances, these can be exercised. Much of the attention will be directed to changes in the law introduced by the British Parliament. But young people in Britain are also citizens of the European Union. The European dimension of rights and entitlements will, therefore, also be used as we begin to codify the sorts of rights to which young people may legitimately lay claim.

The changing legal context of youth citizenship

Two major arenas of debate will be reviewed in this chapter. The first is concerned with the welfare of children and young people in the widest sense. This involves the ways in which they have claims to be looked after, need to be supported and cared for, and require that their dependency on others (and especially members of their family) is not abused. This has most recently been the subject of legislation through the Children Act 1989. As we will see, the Act is wide-ranging in its coverage, including within its domain 12 parts covering different spheres of welfare provision, 15 schedules, 108 sections, and 10 volumes of *Guidance and regulations* issued by the Department of Health to direct its implementation. The Act covers a myriad of different rights, duties, obligations and exhortations to good practice concerning everything from: child abuse and child protection; adoption and private fostering; service provision for children with special needs and disabilities; the running of institutions, including children's homes, secure accommodation and independent schools; child minding; establishing paternity; to how a child might change its name or its legal guardian. The Children Act 1989, involved both the codification and revision of previous legislation about children, and the most far-reaching review of legislation concerning children in living memory (Parton 1991). In doing all this, the Act is important in defining the rights and responsibilities of parents, children and young people, social workers, local authorities, institutions catering for the young (including nurseries, day care facilities, schools and children's homes), and the powers of the courts. Above all, the Act is the latest, but certainly the most comprehensive, attempt to bring public law to bear upon the regulation of private families. The interest of this chapter is not to give a detailed account of all the provisions of the Act but to outline some of its main principles and its *potential* for the development of young people's rights. This should not be read as implying that the author has a naïve belief that this potential will be fully realized at a stroke. Indeed, the failure of some institutions to comply fully with the *Guidance and regulations* which accompanied the Act will be critically reviewed in subsequent chapters. The Act does, however, offer a rare opportunity to examine the interface between the private life of families and a legal perception of the public duty to scrutinize and regulate this in the best interests of children and young people, their parents and the wider community. It is also illuminating in offering insights into the sorts of *reasonable claims (and rights)* young people can have, and can make, on the family and the state. The discussion of the Children Act 1989 thus helps to focus attention on how young people are accorded the rights of citizenship, how these are protected by law, and how the welfare of children and young people are conceived of by the law. In this sense the discussion of The Children Act 1989, will focus on *the processes of inclusion within citizenship* and the legal means through which young people are granted legal, political, and social rights as citizens.

Yet, as was argued in the last chapter, there is another side to the battle for citizenship in which people are denied rights and privileges and are limited in their ability to exercise them. In this sense, they are prevented from achieving full citizenship by laws which constrain their freedoms and behaviours through *processes of exclusion*. Nowhere does this most obviously take place than in the criminal law. The discussion of the legal basis of rights based on the Children Act 1989 will, therefore, be balanced by a discussion of The Criminal Justice Act 1991. Since the passage of the latter Act, we have seen further Criminal Justice Acts which have introduced tougher regimes within the procedures of the courts and the treatment of offenders. Nevertheless, the 1991 Act remains a watershed in attempting to regulate the relationship between young people, their families and the community, and it is for this reason that we concentrate upon it here. While it is true that the subsequent 1993 and 1994 Acts give further powers to the police and to the courts in dealing with young offenders, the 1991 Act remains crucially important in regulating the responsibilities of parents for the behaviour of young people.

The Children Act 1989

Parton has described the Children Act 1989 as "constructing a new consensus, . . . a new set of balances related to the respective roles and responsibilities of the state and the family in the upbringing of children" (Parton 1991: 148). The Children Act 1989 followed in the wake of the Short Report 1985, an inquiry into children in care and child care law which, in part, led to the 1987 White Paper *The law on child care and family services* (DHSS 1985, DHSS 1987). The Children Act 1989 was heavily influenced by public concern about child abuse, especially in the wake of the so-called "Cleveland Affair", which resulted in a major inquiry by Mrs Justice Butler-Sloss which took place while the Bill was before Parliament. The Cleveland Affair arose as a result of a steep rise in the numbers of children being separated from their parents after suspicion of child sexual abuse (Bell 1988, Butler-Sloss 1988, Campbell 1988). It involved allegations of mistaken diagnosis of sexual abuse, disputes between different intervention agencies, allegations of unprofessional conduct, children being taken into care forcibly and in the middle of the night, and wide tabloid newspaper coverage of the events. This context is important, for while the Children Bill was wide-ranging, most public interest and the debates within Parliament focused on child protection and the rights of parents and little attention was given to other, significant issues within the provisions of the Bill (Parton 1991). It is these, rather than the issue of child protection, which are the basis of the following discussion.

It is perhaps noteworthy that in the various White Papers, in the Act itself and in the *Guidance and regulations* which followed it, the term "children" predominates, as it did in many of the debates. It is continually irritating to youth specialists to find that, within the rhetoric of social work and the Departments of Health and Social Security official papers covering social work, the term "children" is ubiquitously used. The Home Office and official papers on crime and the criminal justice system have, for a long time, illustrated an ability to use and develop the concept of "young offenders", perhaps because they are concerned with criminal *responsibility*. Possibly because so much of social work is concerned with the *protection* of the vulnerable, young people are constantly referred to as "children" and little legal attempt is made to define more accurately the term "older children" or young people. Despite this, it is clear that the terms of the

105

Children Act 1989 do cover the responsibilities of the state for the welfare of young people up to the age of 21, and, in dealing as they do with children and young people in the care of local authorities, they are *primarily* concerned with those whom it is difficult to categorize as mere "children". As the Utting Report makes clear, a quarter of "children" in care are over the age of 16, and of those in residential care, more than two-thirds are over the age of 13 and more than a third over the age of 16 (Utting 1991). The Children Act 1989 does, therefore, deal with the welfare of *young people*, and has much of value to say about the sorts of rights they can reasonably expect, and which the state should attempt to secure.

The basic principles within the Children Act 1989

The 1987 White Paper outlines many of the basic principles which lay behind the Act. First, it makes clear that "the primary responsibility for the care and upbringing of children lies with parents" (Children Act: para. 5a). In the wake of the Cleveland Affair, especially, intervening in the private life of families was regarded as highly sensitive in the parliamentary debates on the Bill. The Conservative MP Tim Devlin argued that "Family life is the foundation stone of society and we tinker with it at our peril," while the Labour MP Keith Vaz claimed that "We all start from the presumption that the best place for a child is with his or her family and the state should intervene only if that relationship goes wrong" (both quoted by Parton 1991: 149). The 1987 White Paper makes it clear that the state should be supporting families, and was concerned that the state's first duty was to provide "help to parents to discharge their responsibility, especially where doing so lessens the risk of family breakdown" (DHSS 1987: para. 5a).

Secondly, the White Paper argued that, where families are in need of help, this should be primarily arranged "in a *voluntary* partnership with parents" (emphasis added). Again, as if to emphasize its pro-family approach, it added that, where the child is being cared for away from home, "close contact should be maintained so that the children can continue their relationships with their families and where appropriate reunited with them as soon as possible" (DHSS 1987: para. 5b). Yet, the White Paper and the Act were responding to widespread public concern about abuse and as such had to address the fact that things *do* "go wrong" in the care of children, and consideration must be given in severe cases, as to whether there should be a transfer of "parents' legal powers". The White Paper makes it clear that this should only take place where "there is harm or risk of harm to a child who is not receiving adequate care or is beyond parental control" (DHSS 1987: para. 5c).

The third principle embedded in the Act is how, and on what grounds, such transfer of powers could take place. In the wake of the Cleveland Affair, this was obviously a most contentious issue. The resolution was that there must be some clear means through which the welfare needs of children and young people can be identified and that, while these could and should be investigated through a co-ordinated inquiry by a number of welfare agencies (including social services, the education service, medical practitioners and, where necessary, the police), the adjudication of the need for any transfer of powers from the family to the state should most properly take place before the courts.

Fourthly, the Act attempted to establish *criteria* through which need can be said to be threatened. The principle argued in the 1987 White Paper was that intervention was necessary when there was harm or the risk of harm to the child. This was later changed to the risk of "significant harm" in the Act. The *Guidance and regulations* on Court Orders attempts to clarify this. It makes clear that "Minor short comings in health care or minor deficits in physical, psychological or social development should not require compulsory intervention unless cumulatively they are having, or are likely to have, serious lasting effects on the child" (*Guidance and regulations*: vol 1, para. 3.21). At its most basic, "significant harm" can be seen to follow from actual or threatened physical and sexual abuse but, as the *Guidance* notes illustrate, abuse must be regarded as much wider than this and may include emotional abuse, impairments to health, or impairments to physical, emotional, behavioural, intellectual and social development (White et al. 1990).

This attempt to define the circumstances in which welfare harm may be deemed to occur still left open the questions as to through whom, and by which means, decisions to act should be reached. The Act attempted to clarify the responsibilities of the welfare agencies of local authorities, the police and the courts. In doing so, it was also cognizant of the difficulties encountered in the handling of child abuse allegations in Cleveland, where there had been conflict both between public authorities and their agents, and between the authorities and the parents of children taken into care. The Act tried to resolve the mess. It makes clear that, in matters of dispute between the interests of different parties, it should be the courts which make decisions. The Act makes clear that it is the courts which must adjudicate on the needs of the child in the granting of "Care and Supervision Orders", as covered in part 4 of the Act. Within this, the Act further tried to protect parents' rights. While it introduces a new "Emergency Protection Order" (part 5 of the Act), which can be enforced by a police constable acting under a warrant, this was much more limited in scope than the "Place of Safety Order" which it replaced. "Emergency Protection Orders" are limited, under the 1989 Act, to up to 8 days' duration, and can be renewable for only up to a further 7 days. Following the Butler-Sloss Report, the Children Bill was further amended during its passage through Parliament to give parents the right to challenge such Orders after 72 hours, if they had not been present at the initial application. In this sense, while the Act was concerned to protect "children in need", it was also concerned to defend the rights and interests of parents (Fox Harding 1991).

In attempting to balance this potential conflict of *interests*, the Act laid great emphasis on the role of the courts in adjudicating between the *rights* of parents and the *needs* of the child. In doing so, three important changes in court procedures were also introduced. First, the Act considerably increased the powers and responsibilities of a "guardian *ad litem*" who was to be appointed to act in the *interests of the child* and ascertain his or her wishes. Prior to the 1989 Act, these advocates *could* be appointed where there was seen to be a conflict of interests between parents and the child. But the 1989 Act made clear that they *must* be appointed unless the court was convinced and satisfied that it was unnecessary to do so. Secondly, part 4 of the Act outlines new grounds which must be established by the courts before making "Care" or "Supervision" Orders. This is of particular importance in that it involves legislation about the scope of welfare to which children and young people are legally entitled. Under the Act, what must be established, before the transfer of powers away from parents, is that a child or young person has been subjected to "significant harm" or be at risk of receiving "significant harm in the future", and that this harm can be attributable to care falling short of *what reasonable parents would provide*. It should be remembered that this focus on "significant harm" is in line with the theoretical concept of need outlined by Doyal & Gough and discussed in the last chapter (Doyal & Gough 1992). In establishing the needs of the child, the 1989 Act further established a "welfare checklist" which courts should consider before making Care or Supervision orders. It is significant that the first point involves "ascertaining the wishes and feelings of the child, *considered in the light of his age and understanding*" (emphasis added). This, together with the wider powers and responsibilities of the guardian *ad litem* in acting as advocate for the child, can be seen to strengthen the rights of the child in determining his or her own welfare needs, and again is close to our emphasis on the importance of autonomy and learning needs outlined in the last chapter. These changes, therefore, introduce an important fifth principle that, in establishing need, the views and opinions of young people are a vital and important element and that, in order to give these adequate weight, a young person may need the help and support of a professional worker. Advocacy, and the employment of a guardian *ad litem* to act as an advocate, are thus defined as a means through which young people's voices may be properly heard and their wishes properly consulted. It is, therefore, a means of strengthening the opinions and desires of the potentially weak or vulnerable, rather than replacing those with a proxy voice.

The reference in the "welfare checklist" to consideration of the age and understanding of the child is repeated elsewhere in the Act, and figures prominently in the *Guidance and regulations* which followed it. It can be argued that this establishes a sixth important principle in the Act. This makes young people's rights conditional upon their maturity and the capabilities they have in exercising them, and represents a significant move away from tying rights to a chronological age. While this is an important principle, the means through which the principle is implemented is far from clear and straightforward. The *Guidance and regulations* are somewhat awkward at times in squaring this principle of granting rights according to establishing the maturity of a young person, with other laws which are still wedded to rights granted at a specific chronological age.

A seventh important principle concerns cultural heritage. Within the *Guidance and regulations* which followed the passing of the Act are specific guidelines about respecting the religious, cultural and linguistic needs and rights of young people from different ethnic groups where they are placed in either residential care or in the care of foster parents (Dept. of Health 1991: vol. 8, para. 1.7.21). This states that "In seeking to satisfy themselves that a child's welfare is being satisfactorily safeguarded and promoted in the private foster home, social workers need to be aware and establish that the private foster parent is aware of differences between minority group children and the significance of religion and culture in relation to racial origin." Foster parents too are exhorted to "value and respect a child's racial origins, religion, culture and language" (para. 1.7.26) and social workers are instructed not to be assumptive in ensuring that these interests are safeguarded. Young people in residential care are also to receive similar consideration, with staff instructed that "Special efforts must be made to ensure that important aspects of a child's cultural and religious heritage are not lost at this crucial stage of his life." (vol. 4, para. 1.122) Further guidance is given about the provision of facilities for religious observation, special diets and clothing, and appropriate privacy in which to pray.

In drawing a number of principles from the Children Act 1989, what should be clear is that, while the Act itself is important in laying the foundation for the means through which the rights, needs and interests of young people, their parents, and the wider community can be adjudicated, many of the more detailed specifications of young people's rights are contained within documents produced after the passage of the Act and designed to offer guidance upon its interpretation and the means through which it can be translated into good practice. These ten volumes of *Guidance and regulations* have, however, a less clear-cut legal standing. Yet, from the point of view of this book they do offer an important signal as to the sorts of rights children and young people may reasonably expect from the private world of families, as well as the rights of young people who are more formally in the public care. They are, therefore, worthy of close scrutiny.

The more specific agenda of welfare "rights"

Although the 1989 Act and the *Guidance and regulations* documents are most concerned with vulnerable children and young people, these provide important official signals as to the welfare needs and rights of all young people. It is, therefore, both illuminating and important to outline some of these more specifically. The Act has considerable importance for the rights of children and young people brought up in the public care and those with disabilities. Volume 4 of *Guidance and regulations* deals with residential care and covers such important service entitlements as health care, education and training provision, and preparation for employment, as well as dealing with the ways in which young people have rights to consultation, representation and rights of complaint. The same volume makes it clear that "children" of 16 and over must give *their own* consent to medical treatment and that, under the age of 16, children may be able to give or refuse consent "depending on their capacity to understand the nature of the treatment" (Dept. of Health 1991: vol. 4, para. 2.23). It is further important to note that it is the doctor who will decide a young person's ability to do so, especially in the light of appeals to the rights of parents in regulating the giving of contraceptives to young people, which figured in the "Gillick Case" in the early 1980s (Lees & Mellor 1986). The *Guidance and regulations* further argue that staff in residential homes "should play an active role in promoting all aspects of a child's health. Health care should include education about alcohol and other substance abuse, sexual matters and HIV/AIDS and should not be restricted to treatment of illness or accidents." (vol. 4, para. 1.95) This makes clear that rights concerning health are not merely concerned with ill health but involve the giving of adequate access to relevant knowledge, and that this is an important means of promoting good health. The prevention of welfare harm is thus recommended to be attained through giving appropriate knowledge, advice and support as well as paternalistic protection.

Positive rights in the promotion of welfare through access to knowledge, support and educational opportunities are also claimed within the Act. It introduced new powers for local authorities through an "Education Supervision Order", whereby Local Education Authorities (LEAs) can take action where children are not receiving a proper education. Not only are the same rights to education claimed for young people being brought up in the public care as for those living with their families, but the *Guidance and regulations* makes clear that, as they "may be damaged and vulnerable they often need *extra help and encouragement* and opportunities to *compensate* for early deprivation and for educational disadvantage arising from changes in placement while in care . . . The aim should be to help all children to achieve their full potential and equip themselves as well as possible for adult life." (Dept. of Health 1991: vol. 4, para. 2.24, emphasis added). The same volume draws attention to regulation 10, which requires those responsible for children's homes to "assist with the making of, and give effect to, arrangements made with respect to continued education, training and employment of young people over statutory school age accommodated in the homes" (vol. 4, para. 1.115). It argues that, for older children in care, education, training, and employment should increasingly figure in "care plans", and that "It is one of the responsibilities of staff to explore ideas with them and to give them help in obtaining information about as wide a range of education, training or work opportunities as possible" (vol. 4, para. 1.117). All this seems to accept the need for *compensatory education* because of the adverse circumstances in which such young people are being brought up. We will examine these disadvantages in more detail in the next chapter. The guidance given, however, does accept that, as such young people attempt important and difficult youth transitions, there is a clear need for proper counselling, support and advocacy. A similar level of support is also claimed for young people with disabilities and special educational needs. This group is covered by volume 6 of the *Guidance and regulations* which applies to those given responsibility for dealing with young people with disabilities.

Volume 6 of the *Guidance and regulations* draws attention to the duty of LEAs, under the 1986 Disabled Person's Act to obtain the opinion of Social Service Departments (SSDs) about whether a person is, or is not, a "disabled person", and to notify the SSDs eight months before these persons are due to leave full-time education (Dept. of Health 1991: vol. 6, para. 9.22). It further calls attention to section 24(1) of the 1989 Act which gives SSDs new duties "to advise, assist and befriend" each child whom they or other agencies look after "with a view to promoting his welfare when he ceases to be looked after by them" and advises SSDs that "they should takes steps to prepare a child for the time when he is no longer looked after by them" (para. 16.1). Where young people are living with their parents, it draws attention to the need to establish their wishes in planning to leave home and to the importance of vocational training and independent living schemes (para. 16.5). In this, it calls for close collaboration between SSDs, the youth service, the Careers Service and schools and colleges (para. 16.6). It stresses that "in some instances the young people and their parents will need independent advice, counselling and advocacy in determining their needs and the most effective way of meeting them", and that "No assumptions should be made about what the parents or young people want." (para. 16.6) In a most insightful and important paragraph it argued that "Although investing in transition may appear expensive, the longer term benefits of greater competence and independence will be positive for everyone concerned." (para. 16.5)

Within the *Guidance and regulations* which accompanied the Children Act 1989, there is, therefore, a clear recognition of the transition processes we outlined in Chapter 1, and the fact that some special groups of young people, especially those being brought up in care and those with special needs or disabilities, face severe hardship in attempting these transitions. Elsewhere, there is also clear guidance given about the rights young people can reasonably expect from public and private bodies. Volume 4 deals with children and young people being brought up in children's homes. This makes specific reference to discipline regimes, to rights of privacy and communication, rights of choice as to how to dress, and the appropriate degree of regulation of a young person's privacy and ownership of personal property. This makes clear that young people are to be given rights to privacy (especially in their own room), rights of association (with friends, relatives and parents) and rights to communicate (in private) with their parents. In the light of a number of scandals concerning the running of children's homes, the *Guidance and regulations* are also clear in prohibiting material and social deprivation as a form of discipline. Harsh and cruel means of constraining and controlling even the most difficult children are thus banned. Regimes which many regarded as crossing the boundary between discipline and cruelty had been highlighted by inquiries into the use of so-called "pindown" techniques, which took place after the Act, but which were, no doubt, suspected as it was drawn up (Levy & Kahan 1991). Young people in care (whether in residential or foster care) are, under regulation 8 of the 1989 Act, not to be subject to corporal punishment, deprived of food, drink or sleep, or have visits or communications restricted as a punishment (regulation 8c). Further regulations concern other restrictions of liberties (such as "gating" and "fining"). The *Guidance and regulations* further make it clear that young people in care should be allowed to "personalise areas of the home that are regarded as their own" (Dept. of Health 1991: vol. 4 para. 1.72) and have access to private telephone conversations. In all, therefore, the Children Act 1989 and the accompanying documents do much to lay down a framework through which young people are not only protected from abuse, but are afforded the considerable privileges and freedoms of responsible citizens in a civilized society. Yet there is another side to the story. For while the Children Act 1989 may be seen to develop a framework which gives young people considerable rights and entitlements within the family or surrogate family, the Criminal Justice Act 1991 sought to strengthen parental control over them, by seeking to make parents legally responsible for the errant behaviour of their sons and daughters.

The Criminal Justice Act 1991

A second important act of Parliament, which attempts legally to intervene in the relationships of care and responsibility within families, and the balance of obligations between the family and the wider society, is the Criminal Justice Act 1991 (CJA). This Act sought to consolidate what many considered to be a decade of "progress" in the response of the police and criminal justice systems to the treatment of young offenders. (Chapter 9 of this book will review youth crime in more detail.) The White Paper *Crime, justice and protecting the public* contained the main arguments for the Act. Several important elements were argued for in the White Paper and introduced by the Act (Home Office 1990). First, like the White Paper preceding the Children Act, the White Paper on Crime and Justice makes much of the importance of parental responsibility for the young. It argues that "Parents have the most powerful influence over their children's development . . . and should help them develop as responsible, law-abiding citizens [and to be] aware of the existence of rules and laws and the need for them . . . [so that they] respect other people's property." (Home Office 1990: para. 8.1) In this sense, like the Children Act, while it proposes to intervene and regulate family behaviour, it only does so after clearly indicating its eulogistic support for the institution of the family *in general*. Having done this, the White Paper argues that "the law has a part to play in reminding parents of their responsibilities" (para. 8.2). "Parents should have a real measure of responsibility for them [children] until they reach the age at which they begin making their own decisions. Parents should know where their children are and what they are doing, and be in a position to exercise some supervision over them." (para. 8.6)

More specifically, the Criminal Justice Act introduced new powers into the courts over the parents of offenders. First, it argues that parents should be required to attend court and that this duty to involve them should be mandatory for offenders under the age of 16. Secondly, it argues that parents should be able to be "bound over" (up to £1,000 penalty) to exercise proper control over their children. Before 1991, this "binding over" of parents had largely been ignored by the courts. The White Paper suggested toughening up the court's insistence on parent control, arguing that

> At present the power may not be used when Supervision Orders or most other Orders are imposed on juvenile offenders. The courts will be required to consider binding over the parents of juveniles convicted of criminal offences *in every case* unless it would be unreasonable in the circumstances to expect parents to be able to exercise the required degree of supervision and control. The courts will also be empowered to fine parents who refuse to be bound over in circumstances where the court considers their refusal to be ill founded or unreasonable." (Home Office 1990: para. 8.10, emphasis added)

The White Paper further argued that parents should act responsibly in limiting the freedoms of young people who offend, that they should be involved in the enforcement of night restrictions under a new "curfew order" (Home Office 1990: para. 8.11), and also be involved in the procedures of "cautioning" and "intermediate treatment". Where courts are concerned about the "lack of effective supervision and control", and where this is seen to contribute significantly to the committing of an offence, the White Paper makes clear that the courts should ask local authority Social Service Departments to inquire about and examine what advice and guidance should be given to the courts. Where such an inquiry indicates that "significant harm to a young person is likely to be caused because of a young person being beyond parental control, this would satisfy the preconditions for a Care Order under the Children Act 1989" (para. 8.13).

Thirdly, the White Paper introduced four distinct categories of young person. But whereas the Children Act made a concerted attempt to introduce a flexible approach to "rights" and to move away from arbitrarily imposed chronological age bands, the Criminal Justice Act resorts to such bands, while at the same time attempting to superimpose flexibility on top of them. The age bands it distinguishes are: children under the age of 10; young people aged 10–15; 16- and 17-year-olds; and those aged 18 or over. After the age of 18 young people are assumed to have reached "the age of majority" and must be treated as adults by the courts. The White Paper points out that, at the age of 18, "Formal parental authority ceases, though many parents will continue to help and guide their children beyond this age, and should be encouraged to do so." (Home Office 1990: para. 8.3) The age of 10 is the age of criminal responsibility in England and Wales and below that age no child should face criminal prosecution. Between the ages of 10 and 13 a child should be prosecuted only if the prosecution can show that the child "knew that what he did was serious [and] wrong". Within the age distinctions it introduces, the White Paper further argues for discretion to be used in the treatment of 16- and 17-year-olds, according to both their perceived maturity and their "life circumstances". It recognizes that "16 and 17 year olds should be dealt with as near adults" (para. 8.15). But the case is made that some 16- and 17-year-olds may have independent sources of income from work (full-time or part-time) or training allowances. Others, it says, may be living away from home. The White Paper therefore recommended that, in these circumstances, parents should not be *required* to attend courts, be bound over, or required to pay fines. But, "when the young people are living in their parents' home and still in full-time education, then their parents must be involved, as they would with younger juveniles" (para. 8.19). In this sense, as Ashworth et al. have argued, the Act both strengthened parental responsibility for young people under the age of 16 and makes their responsibility for an older group, either looser or more conditional (Ashworth et al. 1992). For the most part it is expected that 16- and 17-year-olds should be dealt with by juvenile courts (renamed "Youth Courts"), except in cases in which they are jointly accused with persons over the age of 18 or if the maximum sentence for the offence, if an adult was found guilty, would result in imprisonment of 14 years or longer. For less serious offences, but where bail is refused, those under 17 would be remanded in the charge of local authorities, although courts could place conditions on bail, such as the place of remand (para. 8.22).

116

A fourth main principle introduced in the Criminal Justice Act 1991 was a concern for "proportionality" in the sentencing of offenders. The White Paper argues that account should be taken of the seriousness of the offence, but not of previous convictions or the potential of a sentence in deterring others. It further argued for increases in the use of the full range of "community sentences" for young offenders and increased the length of the sentences courts could impose on young people. Nevertheless, in 1990 the British government claimed that its proposed reforms reflected the widespread view that, so far as possible, young offenders should *not* be sentenced to custody, since this is likely to confirm them in a criminal career. So, while the White Paper contains the *general principle* that "prison is usually not the best way of dealing with many less serious property crimes" (Home Office 1990: para. 1.3) and is often merely "an expensive way of making bad people worse" (para. 2.7), it also argues that "special consideration" should be given to young people. The White Paper notes that, since 1981, the number of offenders under 17 sentenced to a custodial sentence has been halved and there has been no discernible increase in the number of offences committed by juveniles (para. 8.24). Indeed, it reaffirmed that prison for young offenders was an expensive means of increasing the likelihood of their future criminality. Since 1993, this perspective has been undermined by a new Home Secretary, Michael Howard, who is firmly of the opinion that prison works, and many of the liberal sentiments of the 1990 White Paper have been discarded.

Fifthly, while recognizing that the prevention of reoffending *and* the protection of the public from serious harm should be objectives of criminal justice, the 1990 White Paper sets great store in ensuring that the increased use of probation and Community Service Orders should be seen in a positive light and argues that "Offenders should be helped to acquire the habits of stable and useful citizenship under supervision." (para. 1.9) Sixthly, a concern with the cost of the justice system was also seen as important in framing the 1991 Act. The White Paper included the estimate that an hour of court time cost £184 in magistrates courts and £350 in Crown Courts, together with the added costs of the prosecution service, legal aid and probation reports. Custody was estimated to cost £304 *per week* while a 100-hour Community Service Order costs only £450 *per offender*. The White Paper pointed out that "Punishment in the community also imposes a lesser burden on the tax payer than custody" (para. 9.3). It estimated that an overall reduction in the prison population of 1,500 a year would reduce overcrowding and produce savings of £24 million a year (Home Office 1990: para. 9.7). It hinted at the growing role of the private sector and concluded that the changes "will be carefully monitored and their effectiveness assessed" (para. 9.9).

At the 1993 Conservative Party Conference, some of these principles could be seen to be under attack from a new Home Secretary, from the Right wing of the party. For him, protecting the public from burglars by taking the latter out of circulation and putting them in prison was a price worth paying. The 1991 Act was being reinterpreted here as having "gone soft on crime" with too much cautioning and non-custodial sentencing which was interpreted as offering too little deterrence to persistent offenders. As will be described in more detail in Chapter 9, the media talked about young people as laughing at what the press also regarded as soft treatment. Some of the liberal policies in the CJA 1991 were therefore put into reverse in a new Criminal Justice Bill in 1994 and the Home Secretary announced a doubling of places in "secure units" in local authority homes and a £100 million plan to build 200 new places in privately run "secure training centres" (*Guardian* 21 February 1994). Whether this will herald a move back to tougher regimes which, as the 1990 White Paper makes clear, failed in the past, we will have to see.

Other significant changes in the law

This chapter has reviewed only two pieces of legislation affecting the relationship between young people and their parents and the attempted regulation of the rights and responsibilities of young people. Other legislative changes are also of importance. The Child Support Act which came into force in April 1993, for instance, makes clear that all biological parents have a legal and moral obligation to bear financial responsibility for their child, and set up the Child Support Agency to trace absent parents and enforce this responsibility. The full impact of this legislation is difficult to assess at the time of writing, but early indications are that parents who divorce and remarry are finding difficulty in meeting the cost of supporting two separate families (*Independent* 4 October 1994). As was seen in Chapter 3, the number of such families is increasing, and this is a considerable threat to the material circumstances in which more and more young people grow up.

There have also been other significant developments in the law which impinge upon young people's rights as they attempt the main youth transitions. Chapter 2 reviewed the effect of the 1986 Social Security Act which, it was argued, considerably eroded young people's entitlement to benefits. A similar erosion of young people's rights can be seen in legislation covering access to housing. A number of changes in the law introduced in the 1980s withdrew a young person's eligibility for support with housing and the conditions under which benefit would be paid. The main acts of importance here are the Housing and Homeless Persons Act 1985 together with the housing implications of the Social Security Act 1986. Prior to 1985, bed and breakfast "hotels" had been an important source of housing for young people who had left (or were forced to leave) home. In 1985, a number of restrictions were placed on young people under the age of 25 in claiming board and lodging payments, introducing for the first time an age-related restriction to Housing Benefit (Thornton 1990).

A number of reasons were advanced for these changes, not least of which was the escalating cost of such benefits. Board and lodging payments to young people under the age of 25 were reported to have increased from £60 million in 1979 to £600 million in 1984 (*Hansard* 21 March 1985: col. 1004–5 quoted by Chapman & Cook 1989). Young people were reported to be living in board and lodging accommodation in seaside towns (tagged by the tabloid media as "Costa del Dole") rather than staying at home while unemployed. New board and lodging regulations introduced on 29 April 1985 required them to move on at regular intervals if they wished to continue claiming at the same rate. In 1989, the time restrictions requiring young people to move on were abandoned, but instead they now had to make two applications for financial assistance. Prior to April 1989, young people living in bed and breakfast accommodation could receive board and lodging allowances which, as Anderson et al. point out, recognized the high costs of living in such accommodation (Anderson et al. 1993). Since April 1989, young people may receive Housing Benefit to cover housing costs and, if over the age of 18, they may receive Income Support (at a specially reduced rate for 18–25-year-olds), which is now intended to cover *all* other living expenses including heating, lighting and food. Since 1989, those young people resident in hostels for the homeless are also covered by this arrangement. A national survey of the homeless published in 1993 indicated that the average income of young people aged under 25 who were in bed and breakfast or hostel accommodation was only £31 a week (Anderson et al. 1993). All this points to the difficulties faced by young people who are not resident in the parental home. They have had lower social security benefit entitlements since 1988 and the payment systems for Housing Benefit have made it more and more difficult for them to live independently of their parents. Part III of the Housing and Homeless Persons Act 1985 gives local authorities the responsibility to house homeless people who meet four criteria. To be defined as in "priority need" persons must: be homeless or be threatened with homelessness within 28 days; not have made themselves intentionally homeless; be in priority need (i.e. pregnant women, households with children, vulnerable as a result of old age, mental illness, handicap or physical disability or other special reason, or homeless due to an emergency (flood, fire, etc.); have a local connection. The young and homeless, therefore, do not qualify *per se* as a priority group, and where the young homeless are male, they are most unlikely to be defined as a priority group. As with the changes in Income Support for the young unemployed, there has also been an attempt to target housing support at those "in greatest need" (Chapman & Cook 1989). Yet, even when need is manifestly widespread, as it is in the growth of the young homeless, the young, it seems, are not a priority and their needs are ignored by the welfare state (Jones 1993a).

This review of the legal framework has, therefore, suggested that recent legislative changes have been a mixed blessing for the welfare of young people. On the one hand, there is the potential within the Children Act 1989 for a positive agenda of welfare rights for young people. On the other, changes in criminal justice legislation have meant that the errant behaviour of young people places greater and greater strain on families who have been made legally responsible for their behaviour. And as more and more young people leave families under strain (or are told to leave by their parents), changes in housing and social security benefits mean that they are less likely to be able to live independently of their families unless they are fortunate enough to obtain lucrative employment (Jones 1993a). Yet, both the young people being brought up in families under strain and those being brought up in the public care, because their families could not cope, are least likely to gain well-paid employment or to be able to afford to live independently. We will review the plight of these young people in the next chapter. Meanwhile it is important to summarize what we have gleaned from this review of young people and the law and outline why it is important to move towards a more specific codification of young people's rights.

Young people's rights

The appendix provides a paradigm of rights for young people. It was developed during the course of researching and writing this book. It is based upon the review of youth citizenship and the rights, needs and interests of young people, the social policy implications of membership of the European Union, and legislation specific to Britain. The main aim of this paradigm is to distill the sometimes complex discussion of rights, needs and interests of young people into simple claims which can be made for how their better welfare might be achieved. In part, this paradigm of rights is based upon welfare principles which are embedded in such legislation as the Children Act 1989. As we have seen in this chapter, this Act lays down a number of principles about the assessment of need and welfare provision for young people when day-to-day responsibilities pass from parents to agents of the state. Yet, in adjudicating the appropriate parameters of responsibility and in developing appropriate guidance and regulations on how *public care* of young people might be properly discharged, the Act does establish principles through which the welfare of young people should be protected, developed and sustained. Similar claims could be made of European legislation, treaties and regulations, although, at the time of writing, the British government has indicated its intention to resist the Social Chapter of the Maastricht Treaty. Given that we might, in the near future, see a change of government and the acceptance of the Social Chapter, or that aspects of it may prove irresistable despite the intentions of government, a youth agenda from Europe has been added to that abstracted from The Children Act 1989.

Several principles lie at the heart of a paradigm for young people's rights. First, we must be clear as to why young people constitute a distinctive group if they are to be afforded special rights. It has been

121

argued in the last two chapters that young people have distinctive needs, rights and interests which follow from the conceptualization of youth as a series of transitions from the relative dependency of childhood to the relative independence of adulthood. This period in the life course is a time when young people, and those around them, make a number of serious and critical decisions about their future careers, and in conceptualizing *youth* we have emphasized the importance of the concept of *career* to signal the importance of the decision-making process. Young people make decisions – to stay on at school or to leave; to leave home; to start new partnerships, for instance – but others around them also make decisions for them, and are influential in offering guidance, help and support to ensure that wise decisions are made. Young people sometimes make unwise decisions and, as the pages of this book illustrate, those charged with their welfare often also make unwise and unhelpful interventions in shaping youth transitions. If these are to be avoided, all concerned need to think clearly about the consequences of their actions and provide a welfare environment in which mistakes, failures and missed opportunities are least likely to occur. This is most likely to be developed where *all* concerned understand the complexities and risks in decisions made about young people's career development. *Rights to knowledge* lie at the heart of the paradigm which has been developed. Young people need to know their rights, and those around them also need to know the welfare principles which should guide their interventions in promoting young people's welfare.

Youth is not only a period of decision making, however, it is also a time during which young people are particularly vulnerable to exploitation and abuse. The Children Act 1989, was most concerned with protecting children and young people from such vulnerability, mainly within the private spheres of the family and surrogate families such as foster families or children's homes. But as young people attempt the transitions of youth, they increasingly enter the public zones of employment, training and housing provision. They enter *markets* (the labour and housing markets, for instance) with little market experience and, for many of them, little bargaining power. In both public and private zones, therefore, young people are inexperienced and, as such, open to exploitation and abuse. The second principle for a paradigm of rights is, therefore, to make clear that young people do require special protection, and to determine and clarify the areas in which young people require special protection.

Youth is also a critical period in the life course when social inequalities become sedimented. There is a wealth of literature which documents the ways in which the social and economic inequalities of parents transpose themselves into the differential opportunities afforded to their offspring (Banks et al. 1992, Bates & Riseborough 1993, Brown 1987, Jones & Wallace 1992). Yet most public institutions now espouse policies to promote equal opportunities through which discrimination on the grounds of social background, gender and ethnicity is rejected and opportunities for disadvantaged groups are encouraged and promoted (Coles & Maynard 1990, Cross et al. 1990, Jewson & Mason 1986). Part 2 of this book will outline other groups who also suffer significant disadvantages in education and training and in making the major transitions to adulthood. A paradigm of rights for young people must embrace, therefore, a third principle – that of the promotion of equal opportunities for all groups of young people – if the better welfare of all youth transitions is to be achieved.

Fourthly, if we are to encourage and promote youth citizenship, youth must also be recognized as a critical time during which responsibility for, and involvement in, an active and caring community is to be fostered. The Children Act 1989 recognizes that this can be encouraged by involving young people in taking an active role in decisions about their own lives, and in sharing in the responsibility of running institutions of which they are a part. Representational rights are argued for in the Utting Report. In *Children in the public care* he importantly makes the following useful points.

> Children's legislation makes certain rights explicit. Other rights are implied. Participation in decisions about the corporate life of a residential home may not be a right. But to deny it, however, makes a powerful negative statement about the valuation placed on residents by the controlling authority. Encouraging it offers them a status comparable to that of their contemporaries, and is itself a positive preparation for that life after care in which these young adults make decisions for themselves. (Utting 1991: paras 19–20)

Increasingly, welfare is being defined by politicians of many different persuasions as involving citizens exercising choices about how their rights to welfare might best be met. If the political dimension of citizenship to which Marshall refers is to be promoted, then the involvement of young people as *active* members of the communities in which they live, train and are educated must be developed.

It is tempting immediately to translate the paradigm of rights for young people into a Charter for Young People's Rights. This book has resisted the temptation for several reasons which should be made clear, so that the status of the paradigm is not misunderstood. So far we have outlined why we see young people as a distinctive group with rights, needs and interests which are different from those which might be claimed by, or for, young children or adults. We have also outlined a number of principles which have guided the construction of the paradigm and the legal and constitutional grounds on which such principles might be developed. It is hoped that this paradigm of rights might provide an agenda for both the implementation of youth policy and its further development and refinement. In the remaining chapters of this book we will examine how some of the principles of youth policy outlined do not yet safeguard the welfare of young people. Part 2 of this book deliberately focuses on groups of vulnerable young people which provide youth policy with its severest test. The paradigm offers a check list for both young people *and* those charged with promoting their welfare as to how, where, and in what ways the current policy agenda is failing to meet even its own ambitions. If a more comprehensive charter of young people's rights is to be developed, it is important that there is a systematic review of the rights, needs and interests of all young people, and one in which young people themselves are involved in the debate. This book is intended to stimulate interest in the need for youth policy, what the parameters of such a policy should be, and how, and through what mechanisms, it can be better developed. The remainder of the book and the paradigm of rights for young people are designed to aid the start of this debate.

Part Two

Social policy and vulnerable youth

Chapter Six

Young people in, and leaving, the public care

This chapter will focus on young people brought up in the public care and their experiences of the youth transitions as they leave it. It will, therefore, cover young people who live in and leave children's homes and those who are brought up in foster families. The reasons why young people are placed in these are many and various. Some may be so placed because of bereavement, others because their natural parent(s) offer them for adoption, while others may be considered to be at risk or beyond the care and control of their parents. State policy has always been based on the assumption that most children and young people will be looked after and cared for within families. Yet it has also not been able to ignore the plight of those who fall outside, or are not adequately cared for within, their families. The 1990s have seen a series of scandals and increased public concern about the running of children's homes (Levy & Kahan 1991, Williams & McCreadie 1992). Yet there is also room for concern about how young people leave care and how they are prepared for this. In a series of hard-hitting editorials, the *Independent* newspaper has accused the state of being "muddled and incompetent", "hypocritical" and as deserving "the booby prize when it comes to caring for children" (17 July 1993, 13 November 1993). Garnett highlighted the issue in the introductory paragraph of a report written for the National Children's Bureau. "In Britain each year some 10,000 young people of 16 and over are officially discharged to "independence" from the care and responsibility of local authority "parents". For most of these young people this change will have been automatically effected upon reaching their 18th birthday, regardless of how willing and able they were to leave care and cope with independent adult life." (Garnett 1992: 1) Quite simply, many are not adequately prepared, are extremely vulnerable, and do not cope.

Provision for "child welfare" has a chequered history dating back to at least a Tudor Act of Parliament of 1535 which, as Frost & Stein report, empowered the parish to take children who were found begging into a compulsory apprenticeship between the ages of 5 and 13 and, in circumstances in which older children resisted, to be "apprehended and whipped with rods" (Frost & Stein 1989). Perhaps more liberally, Bluecoat Schools were established as early as 1552 to deal with the education of vagrant children. The concern from then to now was with both the orphaned *and* the delinquent, described in the nineteenth century by Mary Carpenter, as "the perishing and dangerous classes". In the nineteenth century there was a focus on "child saving" because, to Victorian philanthropists, children were seen as the most obvious section of the "deserving poor" in that they were young and malleable enough to be "cured". Baden Powell, in *Scouting for boys* written in 1908, drew attention to the half a million boys "drifting towards 'hooliganism' or bad citizenship for want of hands to guide them". His answer was the scouting movement in which young people were taught to do their duty to God and the King and do good turns everyday. This concern about hooliganism, begging and homelessness, concern for the orphaned, the abandoned and the delinquent, has an uncanny resonance with worries at the end of the twentieth century about the young "underclass": beggars on the streets of most major cities of Britain; visible signs of homelessness and destitution in "cardboard cities"; a rise in teenage pregnancy and single motherhood; and newspapers willing to proclaim both the high levels, and vicious intrusiveness, of youth crime.

Yet there has been a century of legislative attempts to try to address these problems and set up institutional means through which to do so. Legal interventions saw the setting-up of: Children's Committees, after the Royal Commission on the Poor Law in 1909; residential homes, to replace the Workhouse in 1913; Approved Schools to replace Reform Schools under the Children and Young Person's Act 1933; and a Children's Service and Children's Departments ushered in by the Children Act 1948. The Children and Young Person's Act 1933 encouraged local authorities to take preventive measures to stop children coming into care, and the 1969 Act, in abolishing Approved Schools, tried to reduce the distinction between offenders and non-offenders being brought into care. All this resulted in those in the public care being a worrying mixture of the bad and the mad, the abused and abusers, bullies and the bullied, the disturbed and the disturbing, offenders, orphans, and the casualties of family breakdown and breakup, all being looked after by an ill-trained and poorly paid staff. Children's homes became the dustbins of young humanity the public preferred to ignore. The Williams Inquiry into the running of the Ty Mawr Community Home in Wales in 1992 concluded "there should never in the future be an institution with such an inappropriate mix of residents cared for in large measure by unqualified staff" (Williams & McCreadie 1992). In this chapter we will deal with an evaluation of policy and practice for those young people for whom normal family life has proved impossible.

Young people in the public care and care careers

Legislative change has resulted in both marked swings in the numbers of young people *in care* (or being *looked after* by local authorities) and in the types of care placements which have predominated. The change of terminology from being *in care* to being *looked after* follows the emphasis within the 1989 Act on the voluntary nature of much local authority care. Following the 1948 Act there were increases in the numbers of children and young people in care to a peak of 96,000 in 1977. The 1980s saw a reversal of this trend and a reduction of the numbers *in care* from 95,300 in 1980 to 59,800 by 1991. Following the implementation of the 1989 Act in 1991, this number was reduced further to 55,000 children and young persons being *looked after* by local authorities in March 1992 (Department of Health 1993, Utting 1991). Some of this decline was demographic; a simple numerical reduction of the total population under the age of 18. Other changes are argued to be the result of a change in policies and procedures. Bebbington & Miles report a constant reduction in the *rate* of children and young people being taken into care from 4.1 per thousand in 1966, to 3.5 during the "peak" year of 1977, to 2.8 in 1986 (Bebbington & Miles 1989). This reflects a general trend in policy: that wherever possible, children and young people should remain within their families. But, as the Utting Report points out, other changes in policy included a virtual ending of care orders in criminal proceedings (Utting 1991). Criminal Care Orders accounted for only 2.6% in 1990 compared with 15.4% of those in care in 1980, and following the implementation of the Children Act 1989 it is no longer possible to make a Care Order on the grounds of a criminal offence alone (Utting 1991).

There has also been a dramatic change in the type of care being provided. The numbers of children being looked after by foster parents has remained fairly constant: 33,000 in 1978, reaching 37,000 in 1982 and falling to 34,500 in 1990. But as a *proportion* of all those in care, this reflects a large increase, with foster care accounting for 56.9% of those in care in 1990 compared with only 37% in 1980. By 1990, less than half (42%) of all children and young people in care were in residential care, and these were more likely to be male than female. But the most marked difference between residential and foster care is in the age of their respective populations, with those in residential care being much more likely to be older. Seventy per cent of young people in residential care are over the age of 13, and young people in care who are over the age of 11 are twice as likely to be in a residential home as younger children. Although young people over the age of 16 comprise 22% of the total population of children and young people in care, they comprise 35% of all those in residential care. By March 1992, of the 55,000 children and young persons in England being "looked after" by local authorities, the vast majority – 33,500 (or 61% of them) – were over the age of 10, and 12,200 (22%) were over the age of 16 (Department of Health 1993, Utting 1991).

Many young people looked after by local authorities are the casualties of poor parenting or bad social conditions, or are victims of neglect and abuse. In 1992, 38,600 children and young people were on the Child Protection register, an increase of 6,700 on the previous year, and of these 11,800 (31%) were over the age of 10, and 1,400 over the age of 16 (Department of Health 1993). Six and a half thousand had been placed there because of sexual abuse, over 7,000 because of neglect, nearly 11,000 because of physical abuse and 21,000 because of "grave concern". Children and young people who are abused can, of course, come from a variety of different social backgrounds, although many will not be legally taken into care (Campbell

1988). Other young people are taken into care because their parents cannot cope with their challenging behaviour. Young people who are taken into care are much more likely to come from socially and economically deprived backgrounds. Frost & Stein quote the Report of the Social Services Committee which, in the 1984 survey concluded that "There is a well established link between deprivation and children coming into care. Put crudely the majority of children in care are the children of the poor." (quoted by Frost & Stein 1989) They outline a number of known correlates of coming into care: an unemployed head of household, or unskilled manual worker heading a large family; poor black families living in inadequate accommodation; one-parent families living in poor housing conditions; and families with handicapped children with mothers unable to go out to work to support the family income. They argue that all these factors produce threats to the stability of family life, physical ill health among family members, poor self-image among parents, and strain on methods of socialization and control of young people in families. This becomes particularly acute as families attempt to deal with older children who are more likely to challenge parental authority.

Bebbington & Miles, in a study carried out for the Department of Health and Social Security, report on the backgrounds of 2,528 children in care, drawn from a balanced sample of ten local authorities and try to disentangle the impact of different factors (Bebbington & Miles 1989). They conclude that children living with only one adult were nearly eight times more likely to be "in care" than children from dual-parent families. As we saw in Chapter 3, such families are increasing in number. Living in crowded accommodation proved the next best predictor of being taken into care, with those living in crowded conditions being three and a half times more likely to be taken into care than those who are not. Children from homes with the head of household on benefit (then Supplementary Benefit) were three times more likely to come into care, while having mothers under the age of 21 doubled the odds. Bebbington & Miles reject the claim made by Frost & Stein and others that the children of black families are particularly vulnerable, concluding that "single race children" from ethnic minorities were not over-represented among those admitted to care (Frost & Stein 1989). Barn too had claimed that, on the basis of a study of admissions to care in one London borough, black children were over-represented (Barn 1990). Bebbington &

Miles point out that, when allowance was made for the other correlated factors, the over-representation of the children of black families
disappeared. They did find, however, that a child of mixed-race families had two and a half times more likelihood of entering care than a
white child. This is confirmed by other, more recent, studies (Biehal
et al. 1992, Garnett 1992).

Care careers

In recent years, there has been a recognition of a need to treat being
looked after by local authorities as a dynamic concept. Official statistics on those *in care* provide only static data about the numbers and
characteristics of children and young people at only one moment in
time. In a major study of all children and young people coming into
the care system in a sample of six local authorities over a two-year
period, Rowe and her colleagues note the "staggering numbers" of
starts and *endings* as children and young people move in and out of
care. This emphasizes that being taken into care, being in care, and
leaving it is a complex process rather than a simple or static status
(Rowe et al. 1989). The authors make clear that these complex move-
ments are not adequately conveyed by year end statistics. Some placements end for good reasons and with good outcomes. Many
placements are reported to have ended in "breakdown", while others
last much longer than was initially anticipated. Careers through, and
from, care are immensely complex. In order to disentangle this we
will draw upon three main studies. The first is the major study by
Rowe and her colleagues which examines what happened to nearly
10,000 cases. The second is a study by Garnett et al. which is based on
a sub-sample of 135 cases drawn from the larger sample studied by
Rowe et al. Garnett and colleagues examined what happened to
young people after they were *legally discharged* from care (Garnett
1992). The third study, by Biehal et al., was of a different sample of
183 young people drawn from three other, contrasting local authority areas. This includes moves *to independence* – living away from
foster parents or a children's home – whether or not they were still
legally in care or not (Biehal et al. 1992). Both the latter studies look
at the youth transitions followed by young people leaving care. But
because of their differences in focus and sampling, it is important to
distinguish between three distinct phases in care careers: careers *in
care* – including changes of placement; careers *to independence* –

some of which take place while legally still in care; and careers *after care* – which cover the fortunes of young people for whom the legal responsibility of local authorities has been discharged. Only by distinguishing between these three separate phases is it possible to understand the complex and, at first sight, contradictory research evidence.

Careers in care

In examining careers in care, two main factors can be seen to be of particular importance. First, the experience of care can be seen, for most young people, to include several different placements. In the study by Garnett and her associates, the vast majority (74%) had experienced a change in placement in the final two years of being in care, with a quarter being moved three or more times during that period. This confirms Stein & Carey's findings, from a concentrated study carried out in Wakefield in the mid-1980s, in which they found that three-quarters of their sample had experienced three or more placements, and 40% five or more (Stein & Carey 1986). Some of these changes in placement are, undoubtedly, planned and positive moves, as young people move to independence units ahead of independent living. But in probably the largest study of young people in care, a study by Rowe and her associates, a quarter of "adolescent placements" were reported to have "broken down" and not to have lasted as long as was needed (Rowe et al. 1989). Garnett et al. report that this was especially true of young people admitted during their teens. Their report indicates that a third of their sample experienced the "breakdown" of a placement in the two years prior to being discharged from care (Garnett et al. 1992). Being "looked after" by local authorities can, therefore, often be a turbulent and insecure period in young people's lives as they are bounced around from one care placement to another.

Garnett and her colleagues distinguish between three main types of careers in care: long-term and stable care placements; long-term, unstable placements; and teenage entrants. The majority in their sample (59%) were teenage entrants. The rest were divided almost equally between long-term stable placements and placements which were unstable. In the study by Biehal et al., teenage entrants also predominated with nearly half of their sample entering care for the first time after the age of 14 (Biehal et al. 1992). In the study by Garnett and colleagues, two-thirds of the long-term stable group were in foster care although, perhaps surprisingly, 10 out of the 29 had been in long-term and continuous residential care. Most of the long-term unstable group had been in some form of residential care at some stage of their careers, including a majority who had also moved to some form of independent living before their time in care legally finished. Teenage entrants had the most complex careers in care. Even though a third had only been admitted to care at the age of 15 or over, half had experienced three or more placements (Garnett et al. 1992).

The school-to-work transition

The second feature of careers in care follows from this picture of change and disruption. Most young people in care suffer severe educational disadvantage. A number of authors have pointed to the educational correlates of being in care, yet the systematic study of the qualifications gained by young people in care still remains a relatively untouched research area (Heath et al. 1989, Jackson 1988a,b, Levy & Kahan 1991, Utting 1991). Jackson has argued that many young people in care suffer a disruption to their schooling because of changes in their placement, little recognition by social workers and care workers of their educational needs, and low expectations of their educational potential (Jackson 1988a,b). In 1984, the Social Service Committee recognized that being in care was an "educational hazard". Despite a study by Heath, which argues that their educational achievements are no worse than those of young people not in care with similar social and economic backgrounds, the studies by Garnett and Biehal help to reaffirm their plight (Biehal et al. 1992, Garnett 1992).

Three-quarters of the young people studied by Garnett had no qualifications, compared to 11% in the non-care populations of the authorities in which the research took place. Of the three careers in care which they identify, even among those reported to be in long-term stable care, more than a third are reported as unqualified. Among the long-term unsettled group, nearly two-thirds were reported to have no qualifications. Perhaps surprisingly, teenage entrants fared even worse, with over two-thirds of this group having no qualifications by the age of 18 (Garnett 1992). Being received into care, presumably, is the final stage of an unsettled period of family life. This, it seems, has devastating consequences, and occurs at a particularly critical moment in young people's lives. These depressing findings are confirmed by the study by Biehal and colleagues. They report that two-thirds of their sample had no qualifications (Biehal et al. 1992). Furthermore, in both studies, these figures may be an underestimate since social workers had no knowledge of the qualifications of one in five of the sample. Biehal et al. comment that "The fact that almost a fifth of the social workers in our study did not know whether the young person had any qualifications seems to add further weight to the assertion that social workers often give low priority to education." (Biehal et al. 1992: 20). Only one person in their survey and three in that by Garnett et al. had at least one A level (Biehal et al. 1992, Garnett 1992). This lack of educational attainment is, of course, of critical importance as qualifications act as a passport to a wider range of post-16 career options and, as we saw in Chapter 2, having few or no qualifications is likely to be a major handicap to early entrants to the youth labour market.

The study by Garnett et al. covers those leaving care in 1986–7 who at the time of the survey had reached their late teens. Only a small minority (10%) were still in full-time education. The largest group (40%) were unemployed, while 37% had obtained employment, and 8% were on adult training schemes. Those experiencing the three different careers in care were found to be faring very differently. Those who had experienced long-term, secure placements fared the best. More than half were in employment and a further 28% were in full-time education. Some had what sounded like promising careers; one was training with the Metropolitan police at Hendon, another had his own painting and decorating business, while others were in jobs in the legal and accountancy professions. A number were taking academic and vocational courses, including one who was taking a diploma in order to pursue a career in social work. On the other hand, among those with long-term, insecure placements, only one was in full-time education, 42% were in employment – albeit a number in low-paid jobs with poor prospects – and nearly half (46%) were unemployed. Of the majority of the sample (80) who were teenage entrants to care, only five remained in full-time education, nearly half (47%) were unemployed, and less than a third (29%) were in employment (Garnett 1992). In the study by Biehal and colleagues, slightly less of the total sample (8.5%) were in full-time education. Very few (13%) had a full-time job. While three-fifths of the sample had undertaken a training scheme at some point within their career, few were in training at the time of the survey. More than a third (36.5%) were unemployed and a further 10% were at home caring for their child. Biehal et al. also report that some groups of care leavers appeared to be more vulnerable than others, with nearly half (48%) of those leaving children's homes with education, and nearly two-thirds (62.5%) of those leaving independence units being subsequently unemployed (Biehal et al. 1992).

Housing careers

The two studies also report on the housing careers of young people leaving care. Both indicate that moving to independent living often precedes being legally discharged from care (Biehal et al. 1992, Garnett 1992). In the Biehal et al. study, one-third of the sample had moved to independent living before their 17th birthday and nearly two-thirds had done so before they were 18. Only 20 of their sample of 183 remained in care placement at, or above, the age of 18. This high proportion of young people leaving care and living independently contrasts markedly with the housing careers of those not in care. In the ESRC 16–19 Initiative study, the vast majority (87.5%) were still living in the family home at the age of 16 or 17, and an even higher percentage (93%) were at home a year later (Banks et al. 1992). As we noted in Chapter 3, when young people move away from home at an early stage, their families often offer them material, social and emotional support, and many exercise an option to return home to their parents when things go wrong or get difficult (Jones 1994). For many young people leaving care, this may be an option which is not open to them. Biehal and colleagues add that "a transition from childhood dependence to adult self-reliance . . . is both unrealistic for young people and fails to grasp the interdependent nature of most of our lives, dependent as we are on support from partners, family and friends for security and a positive self-identity" (Biehal et al. 1992: 3). Yet young people in the public care, although they are among the most vulnerable in our society, are among the first to be required to stand on their own feet and fend for themselves.

The sample studied by Biehal et al. included a high proportion (53%) of young people whose last placement before independence or legal discharge had been in residential care. This compares with only 6% who were *legally discharged from care* leaving from a residential setting in the research by Garnett et al., perhaps indicating that movement to independent living often precedes the legal discharge from care. The study by Biehal and colleagues also reports on the nature of the accommodation to which young people first moved and upon their subsequent housing career. Of those moving to independence, only a quarter went to what was described as *permanent* accommodation on leaving their final care placement. This definition of "permanent" accommodation included tenancies either with the Council or with housing associations, the private sector or dispersed housing schemes. A quarter of their sample returned to the family home, although for many others this was not an option. The accommodation offered to the rest (43%) included places in hostels, lodgings, bed and breakfast, and staying with other family members, friends, or in bedsits. This they regard as "temporary" in that these young people would be required to move on again within a short time. Those returning to the family home were much more likely to be those who had experienced only one placement while in care. Those young people who experienced several moves while in care were the least likely to be in a position to rejoin their families (Biehal et al. 1992). Having experienced a turbulent time in care they were, therefore, destined for the most difficult and least supported careers after care.

Biehal and colleagues recognize the importance of employing a "dynamic concept of housing career" (p. 13) and trace young people's housing situation beyond the accommodation into which they are initially placed (Biehal et al. 1992). They report a slight improvement in gaining more secure accommodation six months after moving to independence. By this time nearly a third were in, what they defined as, the permanent sector, with proportionately less in temporary accommodation. On the down side, however, they report that social workers had lost touch with 12 of the 183 in their sample while a further 10 were in custody. High degrees of movement within care again correlated with greater instability after independence. Of those who experienced a turbulent career in care (40% of their sample had experienced four or more changes of placement while in care), half of these had at least one to three changes in accommodation after independence (Biehal et al. 1992).

Biehal et al. also report that those leaving residential care were the least likely to return home (fewer than one in seven) and half of those not returning home moved into temporary accommodation. They further report that social workers estimated that 28 young people

(15% of the sample) were "homeless" and had lost touch with a further seven young people (six of whom were still legally in care). We must be clear that they count as "homeless" those who were staying temporarily with their families or friends and those who were in custody. They were not, therefore, describing street homelessness or rooflessness. However, eight young people in this group had also been classified as having special educational needs, and one person was defined as having a physical disability (Biehal et al. 1992). Garnett and her associates were also concerned with the potential insecurity of the residence of young people leaving care. In this study, at the time of being discharged from care, social workers reported that the majority, (51%) of young people, had been placed in a permanent home but a further 41% had been placed in some "bridging" accommodation. Two to three years later, two-thirds of them had moved, some 40% more than had either been anticipated, or planned for, by their social workers (Garnett 1992).

Financial support and poverty

Biehal and her colleagues comment on the poverty caused both by unemployment, low wages and training allowances and the cost of living independently. With income support for 18–24-year-olds at £28.80 at the time of the survey and the YT training allowance for 16-year-olds £29.50, many of those leaving care for "independence" did so in considerable poverty. More than half (56%) of their sample had a net weekly income of less than £50, more than a third (36%) less than £30 per week, and some others (7%) reported as having no income at all (mainly because they were in custody or living with their families). A study by the National Children's Home reported that a third of their sample of care leavers skimped on food, including young mothers and young care leavers who were pregnant (National Children's Home 1993). Government justification of the lower rate of Income Support for 18–24-year-olds is based on the assumption that most young people in this age group are living in households with other adult members (Department of Social Security statement, quoted in the *Independent*, 9 October 1993). Yet, as we have seen, this is patently not the case for the majority of young people leaving care. Under the Children Act 1989, local authorities have discretionary powers to offer financial assistance. Biehal et al. found that some authorities did attempt to compensate for the minimal income levels,

with a third of their sample (37%) receiving some "to
weekly income *at some stage.* Yet they comment that '
the picture remains one of piecemeal growth and unev
of services" (Biehal et al. 1992: 24). The other major source or financial support in making the transition from care is through special
"Leaving Care Grants". The survey by Garnett and colleagues found
that only 39% of their sample received such a grant (Garnett 1992).
The study by Biehal et al. reports that two-thirds of their sample had
received *some* financial support from Social Services, with 42.5%
receiving a Leaving Care Grant. The amounts given through such
grants ranged from £50 to £1,000, with young women being the
most likely to receive larger grants to meet the costs of furnishing
their own permanent tenancies.

As local authorities have come under increasing financial pressure
in the 1990s, there are some signs that even these payments have begun to dry up and young people leaving care are being encouraged to
seek funding from even less reliable sources of support. Many are
being encouraged to seek Community Care Grants which are payments made under the Social Fund administered by the Department
of Social Security. There are, however, some real difficulties with
these. While Community Care Grants are payments from the Social
Fund which do not require to be repaid, the Social Fund budget is
capped and, as such, receiving a grant from this source involves competition for scarce resources rather than being given as a matter of
entitlement. Furthermore, to be entitled to claim such a grant, the
applicant must be in receipt of Income Support and, therefore, be
unemployed and not on a training scheme. One study of a training
hostel set up in an attempt to break the no job, no home cycle reported that some young care leavers were very deliberately rejecting
training so that, as they were discharged from care, they would be
eligible for a Community Care Grant, without which they knew they
would not be able to afford the wherewithal to live independently
(Baldwin 1994).

After-care support

After-care support is of particular importance to all groups of care
leavers, including those young people who have been in foster care.
As we have already described, care leavers are in the worst position to
compete for jobs and training, most likely to be asked to live inde-

pendently at an early age, and very likely to be in receipt of levels of benefit designed for those who live in better circumstances. In facing a hostile world with few resources they obviously need both preparation for the tasks they face and support in trying to accomplish them. Help might be expected from their own families, from foster families, from the children's homes they leave, or from social workers charged with their welfare. Yet the recent research suggests that many fall through this precarious net of divided obligations and responsibilities. Few young people discharged from foster care continue to live with foster parents afterwards. Research carried out by the National Foster Care Association (NFCA) indicated that only 5.5% of those who legally left the care of foster carers continued to live with them after care was legally discharged, although a third remained in contact with them (NFCA 1992). Biehal and colleagues report that just over a third (36%) of their sample were still receiving some support from ex-foster families. They also report that, in the opinion of social workers, 79% of young people were in contact with their parents. In the same study, social workers reported that they themselves were supporting nine out of ten young people who were legally in care, but only just over a third of those legally discharged (Biehal et al. 1992). Garnett et al. also report that following the legal discharge from care, social workers no longer maintained contact with two-thirds of their sample (Garnett 1992). There was, however, an expectation that young people would return to them if they needed help. Biehal et al. claim that within a few months of leaving care, nearly half their sample were receiving support from their social worker, but that one-quarter (25.5%) were receiving no professional support at all. Again, it was those who were still legally in care who were more likely to be given support. Of particular concern is their finding that about one-fifth of those defined by social workers as having special needs (5 out of 23) were receiving no support. They do add, however, that social workers may not be the best people to provide after care for all young people. For those leaving residential care, they comment that "given the role played by key workers in residential care in helping young people prepare for transition, further thought may need to be given to enabling that support role to continue beyond care. It may be that for many care leavers those people who were closest to them prior to transition may be best placed to offer continuing support." (Biehal et al. 1992: 25–6)

Parenthood

In the study by Biehal et al., young women (34%) were more likely to move initially to a permanent tenancy than young men (17%); much more likely to have moved to independence from foster care; and more likely to have made use of independence units. This was at least in part explained by 20 young women, nearly a quarter of the female sample in "permanent" accommodation, having children. Twenty-three young people (13% of the sample) were parents at the time of their survey, with 20 of these (all young women and 23% of the female sample) living with their children. This compares with only 4% of young women with children as reported in the ESRC 16–19 Initiative study of a more general population (Banks et al. 1992). In the study of care leavers by Biehal et al., 8 of the 20 young women with a child were single mothers. Four-fifths of young mothers had no qualifications and none were in either full-time employment or education. Well over three-quarters of them had secured tenancies compared with only a quarter of those without children. Garnett and colleagues also report roughly the same instance of teenage pregnancies and early motherhood, with one in seven of their female care leavers either a parent or pregnant at the time of leaving care (Garnett 1992). These findings go some way to substantiating the fact that, not only are young people leaving care expected to live independently at an earlier age than those not in care, but that they take on the responsibilities of parenting at an earlier age and often do so under severe hardship.

The impact of the Children Act 1989

As we saw in Chapter 5, the response of the Children Act 1989 was an attempt both to reduce the numbers of children and young people being taken into public care and to make certain that their needs were properly addressed should they need to be looked after by local authorities. Policy was thus first directed towards support for families so that, as far as possible, they could be kept together. Should young people be looked after by local authorities, policies were directed towards the reuniting of families wherever possible. When in public care, the welfare of children and young people was to be properly addressed, including the provision of adequate preparation for leaving care. Much of the research that has so far been reviewed in this chapter took place ahead of the full implementation of the 1989 Act. What remains in doubt is whether the bold aims of the Act, and the *Guidance and regulations* given by the Department of Health for its implementation, are in fact being fulfilled. It is to this evaluation of policy implementation that we now turn.

Residential care

Biehal and her colleagues argue that "residential care is a placement experience at some stage by a majority of young people in the care system", reporting that nearly two-thirds of their sample had experienced at least one placement in a children's home. Given this, they argue that residential care should "have a recognized status equivalent to that of foster care and a level of resourcing that will enable a quality of service to be made available to teenagers preparing to move into the adult world" (Biehal et al. 1992). Yet at the beginning of the 1990s, there were a number of reports on residential care, many of them highly critical of the regimes of control used and reporting widespread abuse against young people (Levy & Kahan 1991, Utting 1991, Wagner 1992). Despite such powerful and widespread condemnation of the running of children's homes in the past, the Utting Report, while welcoming a reduction of the numbers of children and young people being looked after in residential care, still argues that there is a need for residential provision (Utting 1991). Both this report and that by Wagner in 1992 agree that such provision is necessary: for those young people who have decided not to be fostered; for those who have had bad experiences of foster care; for those who have been abused within families; where a family placement is deemed inappropriate; or for those in situations where families cannot be kept together (Utting 1991, Wagner 1992). They did, however, agree that there should be a clearer system to help ensure *appropriate* placement. The range of provisions is, as Utting points out, a "bewildering variety of residential institutions" including community homes maintained or assisted by local authorities (which account for 80% of residential placements), voluntary homes and hostels, private homes, boarding schools (both maintained and independent), NHS hospitals and units, mental nursing homes and penal institutions. Six local authorities in England have no homes for which they are directly responsible, preferring instead to buy in provision from either the voluntary or private sectors or from other areas. But the majority of local authorities do make some provision of their own for residential care (Department of Health 1993).

Current government thinking on residential care for young people is represented by the two reports already mentioned together with volume 4 of the Children Act 1989, *Guidance and regulations* (Department of Health 1991: vol. 4, Utting 1991, Wagner 1992). These documents seem to accept a number of basic principles: there should be a range of different types of provision; homes should be guided by the idea that "small is beautiful" and attempt to give due regard to privacy, self-esteem, social and emotional development and progression beyond care; staff should be properly recruited, screened, trained, supervised and managed; residents should be given proper consultation and mechanisms for complaint; homes should be effectively inspected and their running closely monitored; and finally, that all homes should have clearly defined purposes and objectives. The Utting Report recommends that, in the reshaping of residential provision, "the purpose of the establishment and the objectives for individual young people should be clear" (Utting 1991: para. 2.28). What is also made clear by both the Utting and Wagner Reports is that there is still a multiplicity of functions being required of residential care for young people: from respite care to after-care support for former residents; preparatory care for those moving either to other placements or independent living; secure accommodation for those in need of care and control; and therapeutic care for those who are socially or emotionally damaged (Utting 1991, Wagner 1992).

The Department of Health (DoH) accepted the recommendation of the Utting Report that the implementation of the Children Act should be closely monitored. Regulation 4 of the Children Act 1989 makes clear that all homes should have a written statement on the purpose of the home which would describe to those working there, and to parents, young people, and those responsible for arranging placements, the specific aims and objectives of each home. Clearly defined purposes and objectives are important, therefore, to inform staff properly about the running of the home and to enable appropriate placements to be made to it. Local authorities were required to draw up written statements on these matters by 14 January 1992. Yet, in a survey conducted for the DoH in June 1992, just under half of all local authorities had failed to do so. Some were still trying to complete the process. But the 1993 report on the implementation of the Children Act concluded, "It is of considerable concern, however, that eighteen authorities appeared to have taken no action whatsoever on this requirement. This raises the question of whether these authorities have sound strategies for child care generally and for residential care in particular." (DoH 1993: para. 5.12) As we outlined in Chapter 5, volume 4 of the *Guidance and regulations* also makes specific requirements and recommendations about the running of residential homes. Local authorities are required to give specific guidance to staff on such matters as: working with children of the opposite sex; being alert to the risks of abuse; disciplinary measures within homes; dealing with aggression, violence and challenging behaviour; regulating and vetting visitors; keeping a diary and logbook of significant events; and working with parents. Following the acceptance of the recommendations of the Utting Report, local authorities were further required to have regular monthly reports of a visit from an "arm's length" independent inspector, preferably a member of the Local Authority Social Service Committee. Further guidance was given about the facilities to be made available in children's homes, and the development of "care plans" for all young people in care and which must include preparation for leaving care. All this is clearly important in the securing of young people's rights and in meeting their needs. Yet the survey conducted for the DoH in June 1992 suggests that implementation of these requirements has been patchy and slow. Eight authorities had issued guidance on *none* of the key seven requirements identified by the DoH, and a further 13 had issued guidance on only one of them. Despite widespread public concern about sexual abuse in children's homes following the Beck Inquiry, only 70 of the 104 authorities had issued guidance on sexual abuse as required by regulation 19 of the *Guidance and regulations*. The fact that 34 had not done so is reported by the DoH as "a matter for concern" (DoH 1993: para. 5.19). The survey also found that 62 authorities had not issued guidance to staff working with members of the opposite sex (para. 5.17). And while 92 local authorities had complied with the instructions on approved sanctions and disciplinary measures, 11 had not done so, and 5 refused to answer the question. Another of the recommendations of the Utting Report accepted in the *Guidance and regulations* concerned the regular and frequent inspection of homes. This is, in part, a means through which the interests of young people can be continually guaranteed. Yet the 1992 survey indicates that more than half of all local authorities were failing to comply with the recommendations (DoH 1993). Clearly, these authorities were flouting the law. Other points made in the *Guidance and regulations* advise on good practice rather than set legal requirements. The provision of publicly available telephones which afford young people private access to the world outside is argued for by the Utting Report (Utting 1991), and volume 4 of the *Guidance and regulations* also calls for this, pointing to the need to establish "help lines". Yet, as the 1992 survey revealed, less than half of all authorities had complied "fully" or "largely" with this requirement. The report comments that this "raises the question whether the reasons are cost, professional objections, or managerial inactivity. What is worrying is the possibility that failure to install telephones may indicate a custodial attitude towards children in residential care." (DoH 1993: para. 5.24)

Volume 4 of the *Guidance and regulations* makes clear the "duty of authorities to advise, assist and befriend every child they are looking after with a view to promoting their welfare when they cease to be looked after" (DoH 1991: vol. 4, para. 7.1). The 1993 report on the 1989 Children Act draws a distinction between two important responsibilities, distinguishing between *"the duty to prepare"* for leaving care (para. 7.6), and *"aftercare"* support (para. 7.1). The "duty to prepare" is said to apply to all children irrespective of age or length of placement (para. 7.6) and should be part of the *care plans* drawn up for each and every child (DoH 1991: vol. 4). Yet a survey conducted in the summer of 1992, commissioned by the DoH and undertaken by First Key (the National Leaving Care Advisory Service), found that only 50% of authorities had developed written policies on preparation for leaving care, with a further 19% obliquely reporting that such work was "in hand". This leaves 35 local authorities in England with no developed and written policies on the preparation of young people for leaving care. The DoH report comments that "the fact that staff in half the authorities in the country did not have a clear framework within which to develop consistent and effective preparation programmes is a cause for concern" (DoH 1993: para. 7.8).

More specifically, as we saw in previous sections, local authorities are empowered to offer financial support to young people leaving their care in the form of "Care Grants". Nearly all local authorities are reported to have set up such schemes but, as the DoH report indicates, there are wide-ranging differences between authorities, with maximum payments varying between £63 and £2,000 for individual children. The national average is reported to be £731 (DoH 1993). Whether this is adequate to meet their needs is not commented upon. Clearly, different young people will have different needs, and the report draws attention to the fact that the special needs of particular groups (young people with disabilities, those who are pregnant or have young babies, those with a range of cultural, racial and linguistic backgrounds) should be taken into account. Yet evidence from the survey by Biehal et al., quoted earlier, casts serious doubt upon whether such needs are being adequately addressed (Biehal et al. 1992).

A similar recalcitrance can be seen to occur in the development of written policies on the provision of "after-care" support. Half the authorities in the DoH survey were reported to have completed these and 20% to be still working on them. This again leaves around 30% of local authorities who are doing nothing to implement policies advocated by, and required under, the 1989 Act. The Act recommends that Social Service Departments (SSDs) should draw up written agreements with other agencies for the delivery of special services such as housing, education and careers education and guidance. A third of the authorities replying to the 1992 First Key survey had no such partnership agreements. This is a particularly contentious issue, for under the 1989 Act, while SSDs can make requests for help from partnership agencies, these agencies must respond only where doing so does not infringe their other statutory duties. This makes housing provision for young people particularly problematic. As we saw in Chapter 5, housing authorities are not required to consider young single people a priority group. Some authorities are, therefore, refusing to meet requests from SSDs because it is seen to conflict with their statutory duties under the Housing Act 1985. The provision of services and resources from all agencies is under tight budgetary constraint, and in such circumstances the needs of young people may be undermined by the lack of resources to meet these needs.

We argue in the Appendix that one of the most fundamental rights which young people should be able to claim is a right to knowledge, including knowledge of what their rights are. If young people in care do not know what their entitlements are, or what treatment they should or should not receive, there is a much greater chance of their being deprived or abused. Yet the 1992 survey for the DoH revealed that only one-fifth of local authorities had developed specific information packs for young people, while a further one-third claimed to have their preparation "in hand" (DoH 1993). This leaves half the authorities in Britain not fulfilling the "knowledge rights" of young people in care.

Getting our act together

This chapter has reviewed the current state of our knowledge about young people being looked after by local authorities. It has concentrated on the three major transition processes of youth and careers in, and from, care. The last section also reviewed how the Children Act 1989 had made a wide-ranging attempt to reform the care system and what local authorities had done to implement these reforms. We have highlighted some glaring failures of local authorities to implement government policy. Given these, it is odd to find complacency in the introduction to the first review of progress towards its implementation by the Secretary of State for Health and the Secretary of State for Wales who choose to applaud the "solid achievements" and confidence "that further progress . . . will be made" (DoH 1993: iv). We consider that the evidence of the report suggests that it is high time that local authorities got their act together to protect the rights of young people in care. There are five areas of urgent concern.

First, young people being looked after by local authorities are seriously and severely suffering from educational disadvantage. The Children Act 1989, *Guidance and regulations* allude to the importance of compensatory education, support and encouragement. In that, little concrete appears to be being done, young people leaving care continue to be severely handicapped in attempting the school-to-work transition. Secondly, on these grounds alone, it can be argued that young people leaving care are a highly vulnerable and disadvantaged group. Yet they are required to move from environments of support to independent living at a much earlier age than their contemporaries and with parsimonious financial, social and emotional assistance. As a result they suffer from poverty, poor diets, homelessness, unemployment and social isolation. Thirdly, despite being among the most vulnerable young people in Britain, they are often

147

kept ignorant about their rights. If their welfare is to be secured, young people in, and leaving, care must be informed clearly and precisely about their rights, and if necessary given support in taking action to ensure that local authorities do not infringe them. Authorities who either do not inform young people of these rights, or infringe them must be called to task. Young people have rights to knowledge which are being abused by the failure to implement fully the Children Act 1989. They suffer the costs of this failure with experiences such as early pregnancy and abuse. They, and their parents and guardians, have the right to know the aims and objectives of regimes of care which claim to be acting in their best interests. These rights must be ensured by the proper implementation of the Act, and the proper resourcing of local authorities to empower them to implement it. Fourthly, young people in care *have* representational rights, and the right to know of the existence of these. They have rights to take part in decisions being made about their future, rights of representation in the running of institutions of which they are a part, and rights of complaint against mistreatment. These need to be clearly spelled out, implemented and sustained by proper levels of support and resources. Finally, young people in care have the right to be protected from all forms of abuse; physical, sexual, emotional and material. Public authorities must ensure that these rights are not infringed. Appropriate safeguards must be built into the recruitment, screening, training and support of those employed to look after young people in public and private care. These safeguards should be extended to cover protection in all forms of residential care, education, training and employment. Only when these and other issues have been adequately addressed can it be claimed that the 1989 Act is really working for the better welfare of young people in the public care.

Chapter Seven

Young people with special needs and disabilities

This chapter will focus on young people with disabilities and other "special needs" groups. As we shall see, considering these groups together is far from being uncomplicated or straightforward. Yet recent social policy legislation does attempt to deal with the welfare of all young people with special needs, and the Children Act 1989, in particular, claims to address the need for policy co-ordination in the areas of education, health, employment and social services so as to serve better the needs of all young people. This chapter will examine the ways in which policy and practice for these groups have developed in recent years. It will outline what research has to tell us about the characteristics of each group, and the main problems they face in attempting the main transition processes of youth. As we will see, young people with special needs and those with disabilities often experience prolonged and extended transitions to independence, in marked contrast to young people leaving care which we examined in the last chapter. For, while young people being looked after by local authorities can be shown to move to "independence" at a much earlier age than their contemporaries, those with disabilities are much more likely to have their transitions to employment and independent living delayed until their early 20s at the very earliest. This helps to re-enforce a status of being "eternal children", which is often foisted on people with disabilities (Barnes 1991, Fulcher 1989).

We must be clear at the start of this chapter about the disparate characteristics of the young people being discussed. Here we will distinguish between four main categories: young people with physical disabilities; young people with learning disabilities; young people with special educational needs (SEN); and young people with "special needs" (who may, or may not have, SEN). These groups do, of course, overlap and many young people have multiple disabilities and other complex needs. It is, however, important to recognize the four broad groups as they differ enormously in size. At one extreme, one in five young people have been estimated to have special educational needs at some stage in their lives (Warnock 1978). At the other extreme, based on the use of the Family Fund in the 1980s, we can estimate that the numbers of 16–21-year-olds with severe disabilities may be as low as four to five thousand (Hirst 1983). But as we will see, what all young people with disabilities and special needs share are huge difficulties in attempting the three main transitions of youth.

Impairment, disability and handicap

The most comprehensive study of people with disabilities in recent years was undertaken in a programme of research conducted by the Office of Population Census and Surveys (OPCS) in the mid-1980s (Martin et al. 1988). The main OPCS studies reported on both the "severity" and "type" of disabilities, covering 13 main "types" and a ten-point scale measuring their "severity". On the basis of these surveys, estimates of the number of people with disabilities in Great Britain increased from 3 million in the 1970s to 6 million in the mid-1980s. The OPCS further predict that this will rise to 9 million by the end of the century. These estimates and predictions are, however, contentious on a number of grounds (Abberley 1992). The OPCS survey samples excluded people living in Northern Ireland, which curtailed any possible examination of the cost, in human lives, of "the troubles" in that province. But two other features of the surveys are of a much wider significance. First, the surveys included a much higher proportion of people with relatively mild disabilities compared to previous research. As Abberley points out, if the first three categories of severity are excluded from the 1988 estimates, then the findings of the OPCS surveys would be broadly in line with those carried out in previous decades (Abberley 1992). There is some objection from people with disabilities to the inclusion in the estimates of those with only mild disabilities. It is argued that, because of the low threshold used in defining disability, this resulted in a much lower estimate of the *average cost* of disability. Secondly, the OPCS surveys employed a concept of "disability" to which many disabled people (and many academic writers on the subject) object. Fulcher among others has made the distinction between impairment, disability and handicap, where impairment refers to a medical condition, but disability and handicap can be argued to result from the material and environmental conditions in which those with impairments have to live (Fulcher 1989). By concentrating attention on "disabled people" as the OPCS reports do, it is argued that we make disability into a characteristic of the individual rather than concentrating attention on the failure of the community to respond adequately to differing individual needs. As Oliver has pointed out, in order not to be "handicapped", we all have to make use of some sorts of equipment and resources to manage our day-to-day lives (even where this is as basic as using knives and forks to eat or stairs to move between the floors of a building). As he says, we would all be "handicapped" in trying to eat our dinners without knives and forks or some suitable alternative (Oliver 1993). Yet, where the provision of suitable equipment, or the design of buildings or the provision of adequate facilities, does not take into account the *different* needs of people with *different* abilities, then some people are rendered "handicapped". It is, therefore, unfortunate to say the least if we simply translate these failures of provision into the personal inadequacies of the people concerned. As Abberley points out, the OPCS questionnaire compounded these conceptual confusions by asking questions about what people could, or could not, do rather than what had not been provided for them to enhance their potential competences. If we are properly to address special needs, then we must recognize that people are handicapped by failures of provision, as well as by any medical impairments or differences in personal capabilities they might have.

Young people with physical and learning disabilities

The main OPCS surveys confirm that only a minority of people with disabilities are young. Only 10% of those classified as disabled are under the age of 45 and only 5% under the age of 30. On the basis of the OPCS surveys it has been calculated that there are 76,000 young people with disabilities between the ages of 16 and 19, one thousand of whom are in communal establishments (Chamberlaine et al. 1993). This means that we can estimate that just over 20,000 young people have disabilities in each year cohort. Despite being a small minority of all those with disabilities, young people were far from ignored in the OPCS surveys. Several separate surveys made up the main OPCS research programme and these included a survey of children (under 16 year old) living in private households, and another of "disabled children" living in communal establishments (Bone & Meltzer 1989, Meltzer et al. 1989, Smyth & Robus 1989). Two further "follow-up" studies of young people were also commissioned by the Department of Health and Social Security (DHSS) in the late 1980s; a study of young people with disabilities (Baldwin & Hirst 1994, Hirst 1991), and a more specialized analysis of young people with learning disabilities (Flynn & Hirst 1992). These latter two surveys covered sub-samples of the original OPCS main samples who were between the ages of 13 and 21 in June 1986. Importantly, the studies of young people with disabilities also included a "comparison group" of "non-disabled people" of the same age group so that some assessment could be made about the relative success of young people with disabilities in attempting the main transitions to adulthood. It is arguable that these surveys of young people are, in some ways, limited by the design features present in the main surveys. Yet – perhaps aware of some of the criticisms of the main samples – in the analysis of these surveys, those young people who, according to OPCS data, did not have an "appreciable" disability were excluded from the follow-up research on young people. This reduced the samples by between a quarter and a third. Yet, despite this "pruning" of the samples, four out of ten of Hirst's main sample reported that their disability had no effect on their lives and only a third said that it made their lives "quite difficult" or "very difficult". Despite this, as we shall see, comparison of young people with disabilities with those in the comparison group indicates, as Hirst points out, "the extent of disadvantage associated with even minor health problems and disabilities" (Hirst 1991).

These studies also help to demonstrate that young people with disabilities are by no means a homogeneous group. Nor are they typical of the general population of people with disabilities. In the main OPCS surveys of people with disabilities, women were found to be more likely to be disabled than men. By contrast the younger disabled are more likely to be male than female, with 59% of Hirst's OPCS sample being male. While the OPCS studies classified the population according to different "types", Hirst indicates that many young people have more than one disability, with 88% of his sample having more than two (Hirst 1991). He reclassifies the "types" into four main groups which overlapped in terms of membership. Forty-one per cent of the sample had disabilities which most commonly had a physical origin; locomotion, disfigurement, dexterity, reaching or personal care. A quarter had sensory disabilities, such as hearing, seeing or communication. A third group had disabilities which he classified as "other" but which included being prone to fits or convulsions, loss of consciousness, incontinence or digestion disabilities. The fourth, and by far the largest, group were young people with a "mental disability" which he defines as having "behaviour or intellectual disabilities which were often associated with communication disability" (Hirst 1991). Seventy per cent of Hirst's main sample of young people with disabilities were said to be so classifiable. In the separate follow-up survey of young people with learning disabilities, "intellectual disability" was also shown to correlate with other "types". More than half of this sample (54%) was reported as having intellectual, behavioural and communicational disabilities all in combination. A fifth of the sample had difficulties associated with locomotion, while more than one in five had continence problems or difficulties in personal care. Much smaller proportions were reported to have a learning disability combined with physical impairments such as hearing (16%), seeing (6%) or consciousness disabilities (10%). So, while young people with learning disability are also likely to have multiple disabilities, the majority are not physically handicapped. They are also likely to have special educational needs.

Special educational needs

In introducing compulsory secondary education for all young people, the 1944 Education Act made Local Education Authorities responsible for the first time for making special provision for those who had "disabilities of mind or body". The regulations spelt out 11 categories of disability which included: the blind and partly sighted; the deaf and partially deaf; the physically handicapped and the delicate; those who had a speech defect, were autistic, or suffered from epilepsy. Yet, as Tomlinson shows, the provision for these groups was tiny compared with the special education being provided for three dominant groups: the maladjusted, those who were regarded as severely educationally subnormal, and those classified as being moderately educationally subnormal (Tomlinson 1982). In 1977, those classified as SEN who were regarded as "maladjusted" or "educationally subnormal" accounted for three-quarters of all those receiving special educational provision, while those with one or more of the eight medical "impairments" comprised less than a quarter of the total (Tomlinson 1982). There is some suggestion that the process of defining young people as educationally subnormal or maladjusted may be done as a disciplinary device rather than in the educational interests of the person being defined. Tomlinson found that Afro-Caribbean boys were three times more likely to be defined in these categories than their white contemporaries (Tomlinson 1982). Barton too has also pointed to the over-representation of young people from ethnic minorities in educational special needs groups (Barton 1986).

The Warnock Report of 1978 has widely been regarded as a watershed in the development of special education (Warnock 1978). It established a number of principles for the identification and assessment of what it termed "special educational needs" (SEN) and called for a new approach to its provision. First, it called for the abolition of the 11 categories of the 1944 Act to be replaced by a single definition of "special educational need". Warnock contended that "a child has 'special educational needs' if he has a learning difficulty which calls for special educational provision to be made for him", and was more specific, and slightly less tautologous in claiming that "a child has a learning difficulty if . . . he has a significantly greater difficulty in learning than the majority of children of his age" (Warnock 1978). She further claimed that as many as one in five young people could be said to experience "special educational needs" at some time in their educational careers (Warnock 1978). In dealing with the third category of need, therefore, we are dealing with much larger numbers of young people than those defined as having a physical or learning disability.

The 1978 Report, and the 1981 Act which followed it, are often credited with calling for the integration of children and young people with special needs within mainstream education rather than their exclusion to separate provision. This claim is contentious on a number of grounds. First, the Education Act 1981 made clear that the integration of children and young people with SEN into mainstream schools was *conditional* upon: the efficient use of resources; the provision of efficient education to those with whom the young people with SEN would be educated; and the person with SEN receiving some special educational support. So while the Warnock Report did call for integration *wherever possible*, the 1981 Act provided a loophole for authorities who wished to avoid doing so. Secondly, as Barnes has indicated, the conditional escape clauses did indeed allow many local authorities to continue much as before. In reviewing the number of special schools he points out that, while nearly 3,000 mainstream schools were closed in England and Wales between 1978 and 1989 (10% of the total), only 177 special schools (11% of the total) were closed during the same period (Barnes 1991). This does not demonstrate a major switch of resources from special schools to mainstream provision (Barnes 1991). Thirdly, both before and after the Warnock Report, the exclusion of young people with disabilities from mainstream provision was arguably often accomplished on dubious grounds. Barnes has further argued that, in allowing SEN provision within mainstream schools to be conditional on the efficient use of resources, the 1981 Act continued to allow local authorities to treat disability as a personal deficiency (Barnes 1991). We have already seen in this chapter that the designation of someone as "disabled" often occurs because of the failure to provide special facilities for those with different abilities. Where schools do not provide ramps, lifts, signers or special aids or other equipment, then some children and young people become disabled by unsuitable environments. Legislation passed in 1972 tried to ensure that all new schools were built in such a way as to be accessible to people with disabilities. In the event, relatively few schools have been built since then and, as Barnes reports, few schools have made suitable adaptations for the needs of young people with disabilities (Barnes 1991). For all these reasons, the Warnock Report and the 1981 Education Act did not effectively signal a movement towards the integration of young people with special needs and disabilities into mainstream education.

The Warnock Report also introduced "statementing" – a process through which there is a multidisciplinary approach to the assessment of educational special needs. ("Statements" are called "records of need" under parallel legislation in Scotland.) This is certainly important but it is also widely misunderstood. Superficially, it can be regarded as a means through which parents can request, and Local Education Authorities *must* carry out, a multidisciplinary assessment and, following this and where necessary, LEAs are to provide a statement (or record) of the young person's educational needs, for which LEAs must then provide an adequate service (subject to the efficient use of resources). At first sight this process seems to imply an objective, needs-led, approach to the design of a positive action programme of special educational provision. But, as with other forms of needs assessments, where it is carried out by the same authority which must also provide the resources to meet that need, there must be some doubt as to whether the identification and assessment of need is tainted by prior knowledge of the limited resources available. In a simple economic sense, limitations in the ability to supply helps to determine the level of demand which is admissible. Faced with restricted resources, Local Education Authorities may see little point in recognizing a need which, because of insufficient resources, cannot be met. And while it is true that the Warnock Report and the 1981 Act did, for the first time, empower parents to instigate a needs assessment and give them rights of consultation and appeal over the professional judgements of those who carried assessments out, a survey of LEA practices reported in 1986 that only 8% of LEAs gave guidance about how parents could be involved and only 6% published details of the appeals procedures (Rodgers 1986). Since the 1988 Act and the development of Citizens Charters, there has been a move to make parents more aware of their rights, and the Department for Education now publishes a *Parent's charter for children with special educational needs* (Department for Education, undated).

The implications of the Education Reform Act 1988 can be seen as a mixed blessing for young people receiving special education. On the one hand it can be argued to provide an entitlement curriculum for all, and many special schools are committed to providing the national curriculum for their pupils rather than exempting them from it which is allowed for under the Act. But a number of authors have argued that this will further intensify the pressure on schools to exclude young people with special educational needs from mainstream education (Blaine 1989, Barnes 1991, Simpson 1990). As we saw in Chapter 4, the 1988 Act sought to make schools competitive with each other and publish league tables of their achievements, so that parents can see how well each school is doing. Given that most young people with special educational needs are known to perform less well in formal tests than their able-bodied peers, schools now have a built-in incentive to exclude them, so as not to drag down their attainment scores or their position in qualification "league tables". Corbett & Barton do, however, claim that such a trend has also been paralleled by an expansion of post-16 education for young people with SEN, arguing that "an emphasis on 'entitlement' has brought a wide range of students into colleges, including those whose learning difficulties are perceived as severe and those adults in day centres whose exposure to educational activities might have ended years before" (Corbett & Barton 1992: 15).

The importance of integrated provision in mainstream schools rather than separate provision in "special schools" is still hotly debated. Some have argued that separate special schools allow for a more sensitive positive action programme to be developed (Simpson 1990). Others claim that severe social and educational disadvantages are associated with being educated in special schools. Special schools certainly tend to be smaller, with an average size of only fifty, and they have far fewer teachers who specialize in key areas of the curriculum such as mathematics, science and craft, design and technology (DES 1989c). A number of authors have claimed that many special schools are "medically dominated", with doctors finding them convenient places to hold clinics during precious school time, and with young people regularly being withdrawn from classes for clinics or special therapy (Barnes 1990, 1991, DES 1989b, Oliver 1990). The catchment areas of special schools also tend to be extensive (up to 100 square miles or more) and this often involves children and young people spending many hours travelling between home and school. Not being educated in the same schools as other children from the neighbourhood also increases the isolation of young people with SEN from their peers (Flynn & Hirst 1992). Being educated in a special school does, therefore, carry considerable educational and social disadvantages.

Yet the education of young people with special educational needs in mainstream schools may also be limited and insensitive. Few adaptations to mainstream schools have been made and few teachers have received any training in special educational needs (Barnes 1991, DES 1989, Reiser & Mason 1990). And while young people with special educational needs may be socially integrated in mainstream schools, in the sense of being part of the same school as other children, they may spend only a tiny proportion of their time in classes with their contemporaries (Swann 1988). If their experience of school is a matter of concern, so also is the preparation they receive for leaving education. Programmes for leaving schools were reported by Parker in 1984 to be "the exception rather than the rule" and Barnes claims that "there has been no subsequent research published to dispute this view" (Barnes 1991: 53, Parker 1984).

After the age of 16, many young people continue to attend special schools, though often in conjunction with some school–college link course. In a survey by SKILL (the National Bureau for Students with Disabilities), more than four out of ten 16–19-year-olds with SEN were on such courses (Stowell 1987). Many of these schools will be the same ones the young person has attended since the age of 2. As Barnes comments, such circumstances certainly do not "help them gain the experience necessary for adulthood, but simply serve to reinforce the commonly held belief that people with impairments are immature for their years, that they never grow up, and that they should be treated as 'eternal children'" (Barnes 1991: 55). Barnes further reports than much post-16 education tends to be segregated. He points out that the survey by SKILL shows that the increase in the numbers of people with special educational needs in education after the age of 16 increased by more than fivefold in the ten years following the publication of the Warnock Report. Yet of the 43,540 young people with special educational needs in further education, only 3,419 (less than 8%) were in courses for mainstream students. Most courses for SEN students are reported as concentrating "on life and leisure skills rather than academic subjects or employment training" (Barnes 1991). By the age of 19 the SKILL survey found that one in eight were in "adult training centres", surrounded by the (mainly) elderly disabled carrying out activities "like basket weaving, or boring repetitive work such as packing screws or rubber bands" (Barnes 1991: 56). Many had thus moved from a pattern of provision for "eternal children" to that of the "occupied elderly" in a few short years.

Youth transitions

This book has focused on three main transitions: from school to work; from family of origin to family of destination; and from living with families to living independently of them. A number of studies of the transition processes undertaken by young people with disabilities or special needs have unpacked these slightly differently and focused on four main elements: personal autonomy, responsibility and self-advocacy; employment, useful work or valued activity; social participation and community involvement, including leisure and recreation; new roles within the family, independent living and possibly marriage and parenthood (Baldwin & Hirst 1994, CERI 1983, 1986, 1988, Fish 1986, Hirst 1991, Ward et al. 1991). The Centre for Educational Research and Innovation (CERI) makes a distinction between *phase* and *process*, with process referring to the social–psychological aspects of development, and phase to the pattern of service provision. In examining the phases of transition, they usefully mapped the range of alternatives often made available. If young people with disabilities could be said to have successfully managed the transition then, as Hirst argues, "by their early twenties, individuals might be expected to be financially independent of their parents, to have established households of their own, and to operate effectively within the community in which they live" (Hirst 1991).

It is important to note that, in the late 1940s and early 1950s, many young people leaving special education, including those leaving special schools, did secure employment (Ferguson & Kerr 1960). Even in the late 1970s, a number of studies of young people with mild learning difficulties indicate that between two-thirds and three-quarters of them were able to find a job as they left school (Richardson 1978, Roberts 1975, Walker 1982). These findings are in marked contrast to those of a series of studies which were undertaken in the 1980s. Four main studies will be discussed here, although it is important to recognize that the samples upon which they are focused differ markedly from each other. The first is based on a sample of one in four families who had used the Family Fund. This had been set up to meet the special needs of families in which there was a young person with a severe disability. In 1981, the DHSS commissioned a questionnaire survey of this group. The sample of 934 included young people with a mixture of different disabilities, a quarter had physical impairments only, nearly a third (30%) had a mental impairment only, while the largest group (42%) had both a physical and mental disability. A sub-sample of 294 families were further surveyed by Hirst in 1983 and 1985 when data about their month-to-month activity was collected (Hirst 1987). Based on these surveys, Hirst is able to reconstruct the post-16 transitions of young people with relatively severe disabilities.

The second and third groups on which systematic data exist are the two samples of young people drawn from the OPCS surveys. As we have already reported, while based on the OPCS definitions of disability, these surveys excluded young people whom the OPCS reported as not having an "appreciable" disability. Two separate analyses have been produced from this OPCS sample, one focused on a general sample of 16–21-year-olds with disabilities, the second on a subset of young people with learning disabilities (Baldwin & Hirst 1994, Flynn & Hirst 1992, Hirst 1991). Both these groups can be compared with a group of their able-bodied contemporaries. On the basis of these two studies we are able to examine the post-16 careers of young people with disabilities (including a sub-sample of young people with learning disabilities), only some of whom would be as severely disabled as those covered by the Family Fund surveys. The fourth group of people on whom we can report are those leaving special education and special schools. This group includes some young people with both severe and mild physical and mental disabilities, but it also includes those who receive special education for other reasons. Information on this wider group remains patchy but some, predominantly local, studies do exist. In an attempt to complete the picture of the careers of young people with special needs this chapter will also report on one study based on young people leaving special education in Scotland (Ward et al. 1991). We start the discussion with a description of the main transitions – the main activities in which young people are engaged after they reach minimum school-leaving age. After describing these, we will return to the three other elements of transition identified by Fish and others, which concern autonomy, social and community participation, and family roles.

The main transition for young people with severe disabilities

The Family Fund studies of young people examined the type of daily activity in which young people with disabilities were involved. It should be remembered that, while unemployment rates were high at the beginning of the 1980s, the large increase in post-16 education participation rates had not yet occurred. The survey does, however, compare the fortunes of young people with a severe disability with a roughly equivalent group drawn from the 1981 Labour Force Survey (Hirst 1983). The contrast is stark. In the Labour Force Survey sample, 51% of 16–21-year-olds were in paid employment, whereas in the Family Fund sample only 7% were in open employment with a further 4% in sheltered workshops. There were also marked differences between the fortunes of different groups within the young severely disabled. Nearly half (47%) of the small number of young people with sensory disabilities, and nearly one in five (19%) of those with a physical disability only, had obtained open employment. At the other extreme, only 1% of those with a mental disability or with multiple impairments had a job. While one in five were still at school or in further education, over a third (36%) were reported to be in an Adult Training Centre (ATC). Those with multiple disabilities, which included a mental disability, were much more likely to be placed in ATCs, with over half (56%) of those with a mental disability only being reported as attending an ATC. Attending a day centre was the second most likely form of structured activity with nearly one in five (18%) attending day centres some of the time by the age of 21. While Hirst reports that three-quarters of the sample had *somewhere* to go on each weekday, a significant minority (140 young people, 15% of the sample) were at home *all the time* while others were at home some days of the week. Nearly a third of the sample (30%) had experienced one or more spells of being completely unoccupied and twelve (7%) had been wholly unoccupied for more than three-quarters of their time since leaving school. It is sometimes alleged that the parents of young people with disabilities are protective of their children, yet in Hirst's sample a quarter of parents reported that they were dissatisfied with the provision which had been made for their son or daughter (Hirst 1983).

Nine out of ten young people had received some professional advice on what to do when leaving school. Yet Hirst comments that this advice seems to be very much tied to the sphere of influence of each professional group. Careers officers are reported to be eight times more likely to have helped the physically disabled than other groups, while social workers were more than twice as likely to have helped

161

the mentally or multiple impaired rather than the physically disabled. Careers officers are reported to be much more involved with making arrangements to enter further education, while social workers were most associated with placements in day centres. This is also reflected in the different career paths followed by different groups. Those young people with physical disabilities were much more likely to have experienced transitional placements; more than half had been in further education and a third had been on training schemes. Despite this, only one had secured open employment. Hirst comments that, while they seem to be steered towards employment opportunities, obtaining a job was extremely difficult, and when they did not obtain one they proved to be most vulnerable to periods of inactivity. They had their expectations raised but were not adequately prepared for adult life without employment. Young people with a mental disability were found to be much more likely to be introduced to ATCs while still at school and quickly moved into this form of segregated provision when they left. For this group, Hirst suggests that there should be a more balanced assessment of all career opportunities before they leave school and a rethinking of ATC provision so that it too can act as a transition route rather than as a permanent placement or convenient dumping ground (Hirst 1983).

The main transition for the OPCS samples

The pattern described above is confirmed by the samples drawn from the OPCS studies which were surveyed in 1987. In contrast to the previous study, it should be remembered that these samples include substantial numbers of young people with relatively minor impairments. In comparing the main OPCS sample of young people with disabilities with the control group of able-bodied contemporaries, Hirst reports that equal numbers remained in full-time education, although it should be remembered that the type of course is likely to be different. But while three-quarters of the able-bodied sample had obtained a job, only a third of young people with disabilities had done so. They were also slightly more likely to be in Youth Training at the age 17, with 14% of his sample of this age group being on YTS compared with 10% of the control group. Yet, as they left full-time education, the majority of disabled young people (64%) had no structured weekly activity at all, compared to 12% in the control group (Baldwin & Hirst 1994, Hirst 1991).

The pattern of transition from school to ATCs followed by young people with a learning disability as reported by Hirst from his survey at the beginning of the 1980s is confirmed in the later study by Flynn & Hirst (Flynn & Hirst 1992). The sample here contained only 39 young people over the age of 16 and so some care must be taken in reaching firm conclusions. They report that four-fifths of the sample had attended special schools, but many left school at an early age with nine of the thirteen 16-year-olds in the sample having already left school, and only three 17-year-olds (8% of the age group) reported as still being at school. Adult Training Centres again proved to be the major destination with 35% of those who had left school being in ATCs. Less than a quarter (23%) of the sample who were over 16 had obtained either employment or a place on a training scheme. These were predominately young men, with only one young woman (who was in sheltered employment), securing any form of employment or training. Three young men had secured open employment, a fourth worked part-time, and five were undertaking Youth Training. A further eleven (28% of those who had left school) were defined as actively seeking work but unemployed. By the late 1980s, the plight of a significant minority of the young disabled was little better than that of the severely disabled at the beginning of the decade. Baldwin & Hirst conclude in the following terms: "If employment is a key indicator of adult status, the findings of this study show that achieving independence through employment is an unlikely prospect for the most disabled young people before their mid twenties, *if at all.*" (Baldwin & Hirst 1994: 28–9, emphasis added)

The main transitions of young people with SEN

Between 1989 and 1991 a group of researchers at the universities of Edinburgh and Stirling carried out a study of the post-16 careers of young people leaving special education in Scotland. It involved a survey of 618 young people and was commissioned by the Scottish Office Education Department (Ward et al. 1991). The majority of those in the sample (80%) had attended special schools or special units within mainstream schools, with a further 11.5% in special residential schools reflecting the long distances young people would have to travel in widespread rural areas. All had "records of need", but only 40 young people (6.5%) had been to mainstream schools. At minimum school-leaving age, the majority (57.4%) remained in education, with nearly half (47%) continuing at school and one in ten (10%) moving to special further education. After school, the sample split into three main groups. Nearly one in five (19%) went to special further education, a quarter (24%) went into some form of work training or work experience programme, and more than a quarter (28%) went into sheltered workshops or an ATC. The research found that fewer than one in twenty young people leaving special education (4.9%) obtained open employment on leaving school and less than one in ten (8.9%) were in employment at the time of the survey. Ward et al. also report that, despite all their efforts to trace young people through a variety of different agencies, they were unable to trace the status of more than one in five (21%) of their sample. This is not the first time that anxiety has been expressed about the fact that many young people with special needs simply disappear and are untraceable (Clarke & Hirst 1989).

Further elements in the transitions

So far, we have reported on the major career moves made by young people with disabilities and special needs. Yet, as we have seen, there are several wider transition consequences of the (in)activity sequences within these careers. As Hirst points out, we must also be concerned about "the attainment of the personal and social objectives of the transition to adult life" (Hirst 1991). First, because young people with disabilities are the least likely to obtain employment, or engage in part-time work while at school, they are likely to have a much lower "income" than their able-bodied contemporaries. Baldwin & Hirst report that even where young people with disabilities did obtain employment, they were likely to earn £8 per week less than able-bodied young people, with women with a disability earning £15 less than their male counterparts (Baldwin & Hirst 1994). As with other young people, as they get older it is earning a wage which unlocks many other aspects of independence and autonomy for this group. Baldwin & Hirst report that "the greatest boost to financial independence, for disabled and non disabled alike, was earning a wage. Those with a job had the highest incomes, the greatest range of expenditure and took most responsibility for their keep" (Baldwin & Hirst 1994: 49). In the absence of jobs, young people with disabilities are highly reliant upon benefits as their main source of income. More than four out of ten (41%) of Hirst's sample relied upon such benefits, but Baldwin &

Hirst report that the severely disabled rarely controlled this income and many young people were sometimes not informed of cash payments or benefits which had been claimed on their behalf (Baldwin & Hirst 1994).

Young people with disabilities are also more likely to come from poorer households. Most lived with both their natural parents and Hirst reports that there is little evidence that looking after a young person with a disability increased the likelihood of marital breakup. But mothers were much less likely to be in any sort of employment. Taking into account family size and the partners' economic status, Hirst calculates that the mothers of young people with disabilities were a third less likely to be in employment than the mothers in the general population. Despite having low incomes themselves and living in poorer than average households, young people with disabilities are also reported by Hirst to have only patchy knowledge of the benefits system. Only one in ten had heard of all three of the three main benefits to which they could have been entitled; Attendance, Mobility and Severe Disablement Allowances (Hirst 1991).

Access to income and employment opportunities can also be seen to be related to the subjective beliefs and attitudes young people have about their "self". In Hirst's 1987 survey, those with the most severe disabilities had the least positive views about themselves although, significantly, this is reported to be related to whether they had attended special schools or not. Young people with disabilities who attended mainstream schools were more likely to have a positive self-image than those who had been to special schools. And while in the control sample feelings of self-worth were shown to increase with age, there was no such increase among young people with disabilities. Having a disability was also related to social isolation and being engaged in fewer social activities than those in the control group sample were. Those who had attended special schools again proved to be the least integrated into any supportive community outside their own family with young women with a mental disability proving to be the most isolated (Flynn & Hirst 1992).

Perhaps inevitably, young people with disabilities were much more likely to be in regular contact with professional workers. Yet such contact seemed to be uncoordinated, and Hirst reports that, once they had left education, a substantial proportion lost contact with health and social services. The contact that existed with hospitals and doctors was reported to be competent and professional, although young people reported that doctors were less sensitive to their concerns than they might be, and that they treated them more as "growing children rather than young adults, let alone 'grown-ups' " (Hirst 1991). Social workers, on the other hand, were seen to be more and more involved as young people with disabilities became older, but Hirst reports that social workers did not discuss health problems with their clients and seemed more concerned with family relationships and vocational matters. Of particular concern is the lack of co-ordination between services. Baldwin & Hirst report that

> Once a young person left school the provision of formal support fragmented, was often inadequate or non-existent. Different government departments and agencies had major responsibilities for single aspects of transition such as education, employment, social security, health, and housing. Each used different criteria for determining who required support on account of disability and there were major gaps and discontinuities in the quantity and quality of provision. (Baldwin & Hirst 1994: 108)

Both reports based on the OPCS follow-up surveys draw attention to the potential value of self- and citizenship *advocacy*. Citizen advocates are ordinary people who volunteer to establish relationships on a one-to-one basis with vulnerable people and remain independent of any services they may wish to demand or which are being provided for them. Fenton & Hughes have argued that citizen advocacy can also help to develop relationship skills and self-esteem and so help to develop self-advocacy (Fenton & Hughes 1989). Young people with disabilities need to have knowledge of the services and benefits to which they are entitled. Both reports call attention to the potential impact of the Children Act 1989 (in force since October 1991) and the National Health Service and Community Care Act 1990 (in force since April 1993). Under these new Acts, at the age of 16 responsibility for meeting the needs of young people with disabilities moves from education to social services and, as Baldwin & Hirst point out, both emphasize the importance of the views of service users. They argued that, if all goes to plan for the late 1990s, "In the ideal scenario, disabled young people will be identifying their own needs and making choices, social workers will be helping to identify sources of support, and packages of services will provide a 'seamless web' of provision during transition to adulthood." (Baldwin & Hirst 1994: 112) The disablement lobby has also attempted to get agreement for the rights of people with disabilities being recognized in law and for legislation to protect them from discrimination passed by Parliament. The Bill was, however, defeated in May 1994. Yet the provision of community care and the protection of the rights of people with a disability is dependent not only upon bold aims but upon secured and targeted resources. Local authorities, in particular, have argued that government pledges on the funding of Community Care had been broken even before the 1990 Act came into force (*Independent* 19 March 1993). But before we turn to the potentials and dangers of these new arrangements, it is important to summarize some of the main areas of concern.

New directions in policy development

The research outlined so far in this chapter makes it clear that young people with disabilities find it extremely difficult to obtain open employment. Yet comparative and historical evidence suggests that this is neither because they do not want to work nor because they are incapable of doing so (Ferguson & Kerr 1960, Lunt & Thornton 1993, Walker 1982). Given this, it is tempting to assert that young people with disabilities should have a "right to work". But it is naïve to claim this as an entitlement without being clear about how it would be met. After all, in the early 1980s, trade unionists held huge marches declaring the right to work, only to find them followed by huge increases in unemployment which have left the young and disabled more and more excluded from the workplace.

Yet work and structured, productive and meaningful activity are known to be a critical key to social and material welfare; and unemployment the cause of huge dis-welfares and psychological and medical damage (Ashton 1986, Fryer 1992, Jahoda 1982). The Pathways Projects run by MENCAP have illustrated that, where young adults do obtain a job, this has a major impact on all other areas of their social and emotional wellbeing (MENCAP 1993). On the other hand, as we saw in the early careers of young people with physical disabilities, to direct people unrealistically towards employment careers may be to raise false expectations, only to leave them eventually abandoned to

167

involuntary and unsupported inactivity in the home. Therefore, if we are to make responsible claims for the rights of young people with disabilities we must also make certain that these are also articulated to a realistic policy agenda, otherwise, as argued in Chapter 4, declarations of rights become nothing more than high-sounding, but ultimately empty, slogans.

We argued in Chapter 4 that Europe often provides a source of inspiration for realistic policy development. Research commissioned by the Employment Department reviewed the employment policies for disabled people in 15 countries (Lunt & Thornton 1993). This indicates that the distinctive European approach is through employment promotion, quota systems, reserved employment and compensation to employers who employ people with disabilities. There is also argued to have been a shift from "paternalistic state intervention" to one which encourages partnership between employers, employees and organizations of disabled people. Yet, there must be a mix between encouragement, financial incentives to employers *and* some legal means through which the state can act as guarantor of the welfare of people with disabilities. The European Social Charter asserts the rights of people with disabilities to vocational guidance, vocational training, rehabilitation and social resettlement. Yet it balances this with rights to social security, and health promotion and social welfare (Coote 1992).

Within Europe there are marked differences in policy and practice. One highly contentious issue is the definition, diagnosis and registration of people with disabilities. In Germany, the quota system appears to be properly regulated and to work well. In the United Kingdom, by contrast, registration has fallen into disrepute, and, although a quota system was introduced as long ago as 1948, only ten prosecutions for ignoring it were made before 1975 and none have been made since then (Barnes 1991). Lunt & Thornton argue that the European approach (through registration, quota and protected employment, and employer subsidies) can be seen as somewhat opposed to declarations of rights which tend to be concerned with universal entitlements (Lunt & Thornton 1993). Yet, if we follow the approach of the European Charter, we can see that employment policy alone cannot be regarded as the single answer to the welfare of people with disabilities. Rather, we must seek a combination of employment, social security, health and social support, designed as a flexible "welfare package" suited to individual need. Not only does this seem to be the route taken by the European Social Charter, but these same principles seem to lie at the heart of the Children Act 1989 to which we now turn.

Children in need and the Children Act 1989

As was seen in Chapter 5, the Children Act 1989 was explicitly concerned with a broad concept of "children in need". It defined this category as including both those who would be significantly harmed or impaired should special services not be provided for them, and/or the disabled. This group is, therefore, much wider than either the group of young people with disabilities or that of those with special educational needs. Volume 6 of *Guidance and regulations* spells out the duties and responsibilities of service providers, and draws together their obligations under the 1989 Act and other legislation. The *Guidance* given on the Act makes it clear that its aim is to promote a co-ordination of services for children and young people "in need" across a wide range of welfare areas, including health and development and throughout all phases of the transitions from birth to adulthood. It further defines "development" as meaning physical, intellectual, emotional and behavioural development and makes clear that "health" should include both physical and mental health. It draws attention to the importance of a multi-agency approach to provision, so as to avoid separate and segregated services. This is of particular importance in addressing youth transitions. As Hirst points out, while all *elements of transition* may be interrelated, the *services* which developed them in the 1980s often were not. The *Guidance* on the Children Act 1989 attempted to address this issue.

The Act lays down the principles and objectives to be followed in providing for young people in need and outlines new duties that local authorities should fulfil in addressing them. The *Guidance and regulations* spell out a number of principles which should be followed. First, "children with disabilities are children first". Secondly, due recognition should be given "to the importance of parents and families in children's lives" and "the welfare of the child should be safeguarded and promoted". Thirdly, there should be "access for all children to the same range of services". Fourthly, the *Guidance* emphasizes that "the views of children and parents should be sought and taken into account" and that there should be a "partnership between parents, local authorities and other agencies" in the design, development and delivery of "packages of care". Fifthly, in following these principles the *Guidance and regulations* further make it clear that authorities should attempt to minimize the effect of disabilities or special needs so as to give a child the chance to "lead as normal a life as possible" and, in so doing, should give due consideration to religious persuasion, racial origin and cultural and linguistic background.

Under the 1989 Act, local authorities are required to: open and maintain a register of children with disabilities in their area (schedule 2, para. 2); carry out assessments (schedule 2, para. 3); provide services which are designed to minimize the effects of children's disabilities and give them the opportunity to lead lives that are as normal as possible (schedule 2, para. 9); and, where they provide accommodation for a child who is "looked after" by the local authority, they must make sure that it is "not unsuitable for his particular need" (section 23, para. 8). The 1989 Act further encourages local authorities to synchronize the assessment of children and young people in need. Prior to the Act, a young person moving from school to training or employment could have been subjected to as many as seven separate assessments by the education service, the careers service, the social service department, disability rehabilitation officers, the disability advisory service, and the benefits agency as well as their family doctors. The 1989 Act makes Social Services the lead body.

In the 1993 report on the implementation of the Act, the Department of Health indicates that considerable progress has been made, although the survey asking about provision for special needs groups had a disappointing 55% response rate (Department of Health 1993). Nearly all local authorities surveyed were providing respite care. Yet one third of local authorities still had to complete arrangements for maintaining a register of children with disabilities, and 13 reported that they were not providing a service preparing young people with disabilities for independence. It is perhaps too early to judge whether the Children Act 1989 will indeed ensure a comprehensive and co-ordinated service. What is most in doubt is whether local authorities will be provided with the resources to carry out the bold aims of the Act. It also remains important to monitor closely whether those for whom the service is being provided are fully knowledgeable about their entitlements.

Conclusions

This chapter has reviewed what is known about the difficulties faced by young people with special needs and disabilities in attempting the main youth transitions. Within this broad category it has attempted to distinguish between different groups and to examine the differing fortunes of their multifaceted careers after the end of compulsory education. It is clear that significant sections of young people suffer major disadvantages both within education and when they leave it. For many, the transition to adulthood is one in which they remain dependent upon their families and, in many cases, young people with disabilities become isolated within these, with little structured support. We have argued that this need not be an inevitable consequence of their disability and that there are opportunities within the structure of recent legislation for their welfare careers to be better co-ordinated and more effectively promoted. We have further indicated that this legislation holds out the possibility of greater consultation with them about their needs and greater flexibility in the means through which these can be met. Yet, there is an argument that, in order for these broad aims to be made effective, we must take further action to turn *legitimate claims to welfare* into more systematic *rights* since this might provide a better guarantee of their achievement. It is for this reason that the specific rights of young people with disabilities are included in the paradigm of rights for young peoples in the Appendix of this book.

Chapter Eight

Young people and careers involving crime

This chapter will examine career developments which involve crime, what is known about the correlates and causes of crime and what might reasonably be concluded as to how young people might be diverted from careers involving crime. In the early 1990s youth crime was very much at the forefront of public attention and a number of attempts were made to link the causes of young criminality to the wider social milieu in which young people are brought up. In the summer of 1991, for instance, there were a number of highly publicized riots in Cardiff, Oxford and Newcastle, with television pictures of arson and petrol bomb attacks on the police and shops. Young men were depicted as flaunting high-performance stolen cars and doing handbrake turns before the eager gaze of television cameras (Campbell 1993). An epidemic of "ram raiding" was reported as taking place around Newcastle in which shops and warehouses were stripped of their goods, having first been rammed open by smashing stolen cars and vans into them. After two young men were killed in a 130-mile-an-hour car chase outside the city, the father of the younger one made, what appeared to be, a proud and defensive statement to the press indicating that his boy was no mere "joyrider" but a professional car thief going about his (albeit unlawful) business earning a living (*Newcastle Journal* 9 September 1991, quoted by Campbell 1993). The crash was immediately followed by riots on the streets of the Meadowell Estate in which the boys lived, with the police and fire service unable to answer emergency calls for fear of being overwhelmed by angry mobs of young people. The media also gave high profile to the "rat boy" who lived in a warren of heating and ventilation ducts on an estate in Newcastle, from which he emerged to commit hundreds of thefts and acts of burglary, together with other young and persistent burglars from as far apart as Exeter, Aylesbury and Sutton (*Independent* 3 March 1993, 7 October 1993, 29 July 1994). Many of these young offenders were depicted in the media as unafraid and contemptuous of the police and courts and wilfully bent on pursuing their careers in crime.

In both February and November 1993, worldwide media attention switched to the murder of James Bulger. This 2-year-old boy was abducted from his mother in a busy shopping precinct, marched for two miles across busy city streets, during which he was subjected to cruel physical abuse, and finally murdered and left on a railway line. Two boys, aged only 10 at the time of the offences, were convicted of his murder on 24 November 1993 and the judge commented on "the unparalleled evil and barbarity" of the act. While car crime and burglary are widespread and "ordinary" in some towns and cities, the murder of a young child by other "children" is highly unusual (Crook, *Independent* 23 February 1993). Yet at the time of the murder of James Bulger and following the murder trial, the media was successful in calling into question whether this most atypical case was symbolic of legitimate wider worries and concerns about morality and criminality among the young (*Independent*, editorial 20 February 1992 Barwick, *Independent* 20 February 1993, Phillips & Kettle, *Guardian* 16 February 1993, Sweeney, *Observer* 21 February 1993). In providing details of the background of the two boys after the trial, numerous attempts were made to diagnose "the lethal cocktail" which had precipitated the crime: bad parenting, marital strife and emotional instability in family life; truancy and poor performance at school; widespread and unapologetic petty theft committed by the unsupervised young; the lack of intervention by the Church, schools and institutions of the state; and a background culture of violence and sadism available on video in the home and from many corner shops. This one case seemed to highlight a more general concern that youth crime was so rife and out of control that toddlers and their parents were not safe to walk the streets in broad daylight without becoming the random victims of a marauding violence. Perhaps because the murderers were so young, the media seemed prepared to search for causes in the social fabric in which they lived and had been brought up.

173

This is not the place to examine either the importance of a single case, or the associated moral panics about its wider significance. Nor can we, in one short chapter, undertake a comprehensive review of the current state of the huge and complex bodies of knowledge about criminology and juvenile justice (Cavadino & Dignan 1992, Gelsthorpe & Morris 1994). Instead, some central issues will be briefly addressed. We will examine the evidence of what is known about young offenders and what are regarded as the major correlates and causes of youth crime. In particular, we will review the concept of criminal and deviant *careers,* paying particular attention to the routes into and out of such careers, and how these relate to the legitimate and illegitimate opportunity structures available to young people. We should be clear at the outset that the main focus will be on "crime", rather than on the more nebulous concepts of "deviancy" or "delinquency". For, while crime is clearly a legal concept referring to activities which are proscribed by the law, there are other associated activities which are not legally defined but which refer to other aspects of behaviour which is socially condemned, rather than legally prohibited. While we will be primarily concerned to examine patterns of criminal offending, we will also briefly review policies and practices for the treatment of young offenders and assess the impact of different regimes for the care, control and the education and training of young offenders.

Young people's involvement in crime

The *Sixth report of the Home Affairs Committee* of the House of Commons attempted to make a widespread review of juvenile offenders (House of Commons 1993). In reviewing evidence about the extent of juvenile crime it makes clear that there is considerable confusion. For example, while the Association of Chief Police Officers claims there has been a 54% increase in the rate of offending between 1980 and 1990 (they perhaps had a vested interest in making a case for extra resources), the Home Office claims that there has been a real fall in the number of juvenile offenders per head of population since 1981 (they perhaps wanted to indicate some political success in dealing with law and order issues). Some of the dispute about the evidence lies in a confusion between offenders and offences, with some claims being made that relatively few people (offenders) were responsible for a great deal of crime (offences). Yet this did not fully explain the vast differences in the "facts" laid before the Select Committee. The 1993 Report concluded that "the Home Office should consider how any improvements to overall juvenile crime statistics could be made which will enable more informed policy decisions to be taken" (House of Commons 1993). We must recognize at the outset of our discussion, therefore, that the picture of young people and crime is one which has considerable distortions and conceptual and factual murkiness.

The number and types of crime committed in the United Kingdom, and the characteristics of those who commit it, can be estimated in a number of different ways. At one extreme, based on the findings of the British Crime Surveys which study the crimes experienced by a large random sample of the population, we can estimate that, in the early 1990s, there were around 15 million offences committed in any one year (Home Office 1993). Yet, two out of three of these remain unreported to the police and the vast majority are regarded as relatively trivial thefts. So, for instance, the most often committed crime in the first crime survey was reported to be the theft of milk from the doorstep (Hough & Mayhew 1983). In 1992, just over a third of all crime (5.6 million incidents) was reported to the police, although not all of these are recorded. The Home Office suggests it is useful to group the latter under a number of broad types. The largest group are car-related offences, with nearly three out of ten reported crimes (29%) being theft of, or from, cars. Burglary accounts for a further quarter (25%) of reported crimes, while another quarter (24%) is categorized as "other thefts". Violent crimes account for only 5% of crimes reported to the police (Barclay 1993). The 1992 British Crime Survey of crimes reported by victims gives a slightly different picture. According to this survey, thefts of motor vehicles account for a quarter (25%) of all crimes and vehicle vandalism for a further 11%, suggesting that more than a third of all offences are car related. Although the British Crime Surveys cover vastly more crimes than those reported to the police, the British Crime Survey 1992 suggests that burglary is a much lower proportion of all crimes (9% of the total). Thefts from the person account for 28% of all crimes, whereas, again, the victims survey confirms that criminal violence is a minority experience, with woundings accounting for 4% and common assaults for

12% of crime (Mayhew et al. 1993). Yet, in that only a third of crimes are reported to the police and only one in ten reported crimes result in a prosecution and conviction, it is difficult to connect the vast majority of crimes to those who commit them. Based upon those crimes which do result in an identification of the offenders, we can cautiously estimate some main characteristics of them.

The social characteristics of known offenders

Of those offenders who are identified by the courts or the police, four out of five (80%) are male, and almost half (47%) of the offences are committed by those under the age of 21. As far as the police and courts are concerned, therefore, crime is predominantly an issue to do with young men. The peak ages of known offenders is between 15 and 18, with that for young women 15 (Barclay 1993). Based on a Home Office study of a random sample of people born in 1953, it can be further estimated that one in three young men will have been convicted of a "standard list" of offences by the age of 30, while only 8% of young women will have been convicted of the same offences (Home Office Statistical Bulletin 27/89). By the age of 35, 6% of men will have been convicted of 6 or more offences; 13% of between 2 and 5; and 16% of 1 offence (House of Commons 1993).

Roger Tarling, the head of the Home Office Research and Planning Unit, has provided a review of data on the distribution of nine types of offences together with the peak ages of offending for both male and female known offenders (Tarling 1993). The most common offence is reported as being theft from shops where the peak age for both young men and women is 14. Significantly, although rates of these offences are higher for young men than young women, this is much less markedly so in thefts from shops than for any other group of offences. Theft from shops is closely followed in the popularity league by burglary, which has the second largest number of offenders associated with it. The peak age for these offences is 17 for men and 16 for women. Car-related crime accounts for far fewer known offenders than might be expected from the number of such crimes known to be committed, which both indicates that offenders are very likely to be multiple offenders and that many are never caught. The peak age for offenders known to be involved in taking away cars without the owner's consent (TWOC) or in theft from motor vehicles is reported as being 17 for both men and women. "Other theft" has a peak age of 17 for men and 18 for women, while fraud and forgery have the higher peak ages of 20 for men and 21 for women (Tarling 1993).

Criminality is often seen as being a problem of predominantly male activity. A national conference organized jointly by the Institute for Public Policy Research and the *Independent on Sunday* in 1993 was most concerned by the argument that crime and criminality are dominated by cultures of masculinity (*Independent* 23 November 1993). Tarling, however, reports that the male–female ratio in *known* offending was substantially reduced between 1960 and 1990. In 1960 16-year-old boys offended seven times more than girls, and 20-year-olds nine times more. By 1990, 15- and 16-year-old boys were only four times more likely to offend than girls, with those between 18 and 21 six times more likely (Tarling 1993). So, while known criminality is still predominantly a male activity, either more young women now offend or they are being caught more often. There is even some evidence that young women are more criminally disposed than the rates of reported offenders indicate. Campbell has argued that, if we look at *self-reported offending*, the number and types of offences admitted by women are remarkably similar to those reported by men (Campbell 1981). Doubts exist, therefore, as to whether there are real differences between young male and female offending, despite the fact that the police and the courts continue to act in the belief that male and female patterns of delinquency are radically different. There is a real possibility that girls just don't get caught, perhaps in part because the police and others don't expect them to be offenders.

The distribution of criminality across ethnic groups is also difficult to discern. Pitts has argued that "If a century of sociological studies of crime in cities has any validity, it would be astonishing if we did not find that the crime rate among young people who inhabit some of the poorest sections of our inner cities was not disproportionately high" (Cook & Hudson 1993: 115). Others have written about "the criminalisation of the black community" (Solomos 1993), and Hall et al. have documented the moral panics about the rise of "mugging" during the early 1970s and how this type of "crime" became associated with that committed by young black males (Hall et al. 1978). This relabelling of "crime" by the media was also a means through which robbery with violence became racialized. Beliefs about the over-representation of black groups in particular types of criminal activity are, therefore, sometimes constructed through the media and become widespread. The white working-class young men living in South London who were studied by Foster in the late 1980s *believed* that their black contemporaries in the neighbouring community were involved in much more vicious crime than they were, despite the fact that there was little evidence in police statistics that this was the case (Foster 1990). Tarling reports on a study by Ouston in the mid-1980s of young people attending 12 inner London schools. By the age of 17, 28% of boys with parents born in the UK and Eire had been either cautioned or convicted, while 39% of boys born in the West Indies or of West Indian parents had been similarly dealt with by the police and courts. Of other ethnic groups, those with parents born in Cyprus, or India and Pakistan were less represented in police statistics than their "white" contemporaries, with respectively 21% and 24% of these groups being cautioned or convicted. Yet importantly, much of the over-representation of young "West Indians" was found to be statistically associated with other background factors such as social class and educational achievement (Tarling 1993). While it is also true that young men born of West Indian parents are more represented among those in custody than one would expect given their numbers in the general population, this does not necessarily mean that they are more likely to offend than their white contemporaries (NACRO 1991a).

The 1993 Select Committee called attention to three different groups of young offenders (House of Commons 1993). Most juvenile crime is reported to be "minor and transient" with offending being only a temporary phase. At the other extreme, the Committee did point to widespread concern about persistent offenders, although there was some dispute about the size of this group. The third group identified is an "intermediate group" who committed more, and more serious, offences than the first group and who also appear to take longer to "grow out of" it. The police and the courts respond to these groups in different ways.

Young people and the criminal justice system

By far the vast majority of young offenders are those minor and transient ones who are dealt with by either informal or formal cautions from the police. More serious or multiple offenders are more likely to be committed to the courts, but if the offence is not very serious it is still likely to result in a non-custodial sentence. Indeed, even when the court is convinced about a young person's guilt, many are still given an absolute or conditional discharge for minor offences. The majority (52%) of 16–17-year-olds and a quarter (25%) of 17-year-olds received such a discharge in 1991–2. While technically a discharge, however, this is regarded as the court's equivalent of a caution. Young people may also be "bound over" or receive a fine, which may include a Compensation Order (and can include payments to be made by the parents of 16- and 17-year-olds). The 1993 Select Committee Report indicated, however, that during 1991 only four parents or guardians were so dealt with (House of Commons 1993). A further option before the courts is some sort of "Supervision Order" which may include specified "conditions". These can include a requirement that the offender must receive psychiatric treatment, some form of education, be subject to a night "curfew", or undertake specified activities (such as attendance at a "motor project" for TWOC offenders) sometimes at special times at which they are thought likely to reoffend (such as Saturday afternoons in the case of football supporters). Supervision Orders may also be attached to a residence requirement about where a young person will live during the time of the order. Probation Orders, similarly, may contain a requirement about the place of residence, an activity, attendance at a probation centre, medical or mental health treatment, or treatment for drug or alcohol dependency. A Community Service Order, which may also be combined with a Probation Order, was introduced under the Criminal Justice Act 1991 and is thought to be gaining in popularity, but at the time of writing no official data are available. Where young persons are absent from such an order, they may be required to reappear before the courts and sentenced to custody. The working of the Criminal Justice System has been reviewed by the Social Service Inspectorate, who, while being generally positive about the response of local authorities to the Act, has commented that the intentions of policy were not always translated into practice (Social Services Inspectorate 1994: para. 7.3).

Under the age of 16, young people who commit "serious offences" may receive a custodial sentence under section 53(2) of the Criminal Justice Act 1933. They may be committed to either Young Offenders Institutions (YOI), to Local Authority Community Homes (LACHs), where these have "secure accommodation", or, in extreme cases, to Youth Treatment Centres (YTCs). These institutions have, of course different traditions and histories, with YOIs being developed by the prison service, and LACHs as institutions of social care. YTCs are also reported to have different philosophies and approaches to treatment (Bullock 1994b). In comparing the different regimes, Ditchfield & Catan report that, while they shared the same broad aim of rehabilitation, the YOIs and LACHs were markedly different in the type of service they provided. They report that LACHs were much more likely to provide better-quality education and training, a more varied diet of exercise and recreational activities, higher levels of "throughcare", and more one-to-one help with personal problems. Offenders were reported to be less likely to be reconvicted within two years of leaving than those leaving YOIs, with the reconviction rates reported as being 40% and 53% respectively. Compared to those leaving LACHs, those leaving YOIs were more likely to commit violent crimes (43% compared with 28%), and YOI detainees were more likely to receive a further custodial sentence in the future. The short-term cost of provision, on the other hand, was estimated to be, on average, 30% higher in LACHs than in YOIs. Yet given the differences of future careers followed by the two groups, the long-term costs of a failure to prevent future offending is considerable (Ditchfield & Catan 1992).

The 1993 Select Committee Report also indicated that regimes and treatment in different YOIs varied considerably. Ditchfield & Catan report that the regimes which institutions operated depended, not only on their histories and traditions, but also on the resources made available. The Nightingale Unit of Feltham Young Offenders received a glowing testimonial in the 1993 Select Committee Report. Operating both a token system, which rewarded good behaviour, and a "personal officer scheme", which gave special attention to the needs of each offender, the Nightingale Unit reported a 98% success rate in preventing reoffending. Yet its staff are not specially trained, and the development of special courses of education and training for inmates was only made possible through charities and donations from local businesses. The 1993 Select Committee Report calls for both proper training of staff, greater inter-agency co-operation, and greater resources for Young Offender Institutions, "the 'Cinderella' of the custodial institutions" (House of Commons 1993: para. 139).

The most serious young offenders, committed under section 53 of the Children and Young Person's Act 1933, may be sent to Youth Treatment Centres. These offer both long-term care for difficult and disturbed children and young people, and a secure environment for those who have committed offences which may have resulted in life sentences had they been committed by adults. Those in YTCs include both one-off serious offenders, serious and persistent offenders and other disturbed and unmanageable adolescents. Most committed to YTCs, therefore, are likely to have experienced a turbulent home life and interrupted education before they were committed. The careers of young people being dealt with by such centres have been recently reviewed in a thorough and sophisticated research project carried out by the Dartington Social Research Unit (Bullock et al. 1994a,b).

Bullock and colleagues report that extended stays in such centres can make the difference between success and failure in later youth transitions. Some of those who left YTCs did not have a trouble-free life afterwards. Four of the 204 people studied died – one from AIDS, another was murdered when later imprisoned and no details are known about the other two deaths. A further two had committed murder and others attempted suicide. While reconviction rates from those committed to YTCs are reported as being predictably high, with more than half (54%) reconvicted within two years of being released, many of these offences are reported to have been relatively trivial. On a more positive note, Bullock et al. do report a remarkable number of successful outcomes from young people who had most inauspicious starts to their young careers, and they discuss the ways and means through which these starts might be improved. Some young people leaving YTCs obtain employment, find partners and have children of their own, and settle back into the community, despite the considerable handicaps they have in doing so. Indeed, the studies are illuminating of the ways in which decision making by those charged with the welfare of highly damaged, dangerous and vulnerable young people can be influential in reshaping young careers (Bullock et al. 1994a,b).

The social backgrounds of known offenders

The young people studied by Bullock and his colleagues are at an extreme in terms of their challenging or offending behaviour. They are also atypical in terms of their individual characteristics and social backgrounds. They are seven times more likely to be male, two-fifths are described as "non-white", they are predominantly working class (except for some committed under section 53) and many have a history of truanting from school or absconding from other forms of care (Bullock et al. 1994b). A number of other studies have examined the social and economic backgrounds of a much wider array of different types of young offenders in considerable detail, though some of these are beginning to seem very dated. Three of these involved the study of people born in the late 1940s and early 1950s (Farrington 1990, Kolvin 1990, Wadsworth 1979). They point to the correlation between material and social deprivation and offending. Wadsworth, in a study of more than five thousand young people born in 1946 found that serious offending was much more common among the sons of manual workers, those living in large families and/or ones in which parents had separated or divorced. Kolvin, in a study of a thousand people born in Newcastle in 1947, reached similar conclusions, pointing to the association of criminality with families experiencing marital disruption, parental illness, poor domestic care, poor mothering, overcrowded living conditions and dependence on social services. Six out of ten boys and nearly one in ten girls brought up in multiple deprivation (three or more of the conditions described above) acquired a criminal record. The Cambridge research on delinquent development studied over 400 boys born in 1953 and brought up in a working-class district of South London (Farrington 1990). This study points to the influence of low income, large families, rundown housing, parents and other members of the family having a criminal record, harsh and erratic parenting, and dis-involvement from, and poor performance at, school. Farrington produced a list of 21 features of the social, economic and family backgrounds of 8-year-olds which helped to predict their later criminality. Yet the statistical evidence of all these studies provide an unconvincing "social deterministic" or "trajectory" model of young offending, one which is difficult to square with the knowledge that, while many of those living in deprived conditions do resort to crime, many living in like conditions do not. In a perversely different vein, a senior Home Office official raised a different and provoking question as to why, given the lack of legitimate opportunities for young people to make a living in many inner city areas, and given the low rates of detection of most crime, most (or at least many more) do not simply commute to commit burglaries and thefts from homes and shops in rich areas (Tuck 1993). Yet the majority do not. We, therefore, have to explain the resistance of some young people to crime, despite the structural incentives to offend and despite the lack of opportunities for them to make a living through legitimate means. Furthermore, some young people who live in favourable material and social circumstances are also known to be offenders. Explaining youthful crime by reference to social and economic conditions is, therefore, unconvincing even in purely statistical terms. Instead attention must be concentrated on the processes of decision making, and the sequences of activity and statuses, which lead some into criminal recidivism and a professional criminal career, others to spasmodic offending, and the majority to patterns of living almost totally devoid of any known criminality. In short, we must focus attention, not on the statistics of offenders or offending, but on the concept of criminal "career", together with the social and psychological processes which support and prevent its development, or which help to wean young people away from persistent offending. In examining these complex processes, some criminologists and sociologists have moved away from large-scale data-sets of dubious validity and have employed qualitative and ethnographic methods to reach into, and try to understand, the life worlds of small groups of young people so as better to comprehend why some become involved in crime, while others do not.

Criminal careers

In introducing the concept of career in Chapter 1 we argued that it was important to recognize the interplay of *structuration* and *agency*. Although young people make choices in shaping their own futures, these are made in social and economic contexts which largely determine the *structures of opportunity* available to them. In a similar fashion, Michael Little, in a retrospective study of young people's criminal careers, argues that while choices do indeed take place, these are often made between a limited set of options which themselves change over time as a criminal career develops (Little 1990). One of the earliest and most influential writers who developed the concept of deviant career has argued that we must try to understand the complex interplay between the activity, beliefs and interactions in which deviance is learnt, practised and justified (Becker 1963).

Farrington makes a similar sort of distinction between four main elements in the complex processes involved in the development of criminal careers: initial *motivations*; the choice of an illegal *method*; the development of internalized *beliefs* about criminal activity; and immediate *situational influences and opportunities* (Farrington 1990). These have been argued, by Little, to develop in a series of staged career progressions through which some young people move from minor acts of hooliganism, to more persistent offending, to accepting a life of instrumental crime punctuated by periods of imprisonment. We will comment on each of these four elements in turn. Farrington argues that the main motivations which lead young people to offend are the desire for material goods, status among intimates (friends and family), and excitement. He contends that those living in poor areas have the odds stacked against them in obtaining success, status and excitement by legal or legitimate means. They are least likely to profit from education, least likely to gain qualifications, and most likely to face a bleak physical and material environment with little chance of any sort of employment or a legitimate lifestyle of material comfort (Farrington 1990). Their chances of seeking status advancement through education, training and the labour market are, therefore, severely limited. In Chapter 6 we also reported that young people leaving care were highly likely to live in such circumstances and, as such, the motivations for them to be involved in crime are considerable.

The series of studies that were undertaken at Cambridge, on which Farrington reports, also point to the early development of an "antisocial culture" among those who, in later life, develop and prolong their careers in crime. These and other studies point to a resistance in attending school and to persistent truanting, although both Graham and Rutter have argued that the evidence suggests that the relationship between truanting and delinquency is far from simple and direct (Graham 1988, Rutter 1979). In a study which spans the generations of people living in one working-class community, Foster further comments on the cultural similarities between the attitudes and beliefs of young people and their parents. Both young people and their parents were more than happy to "get one over on the 'Old Bill'" and more concerned about not getting caught than not offending. Little reports the resentment offenders-to-be feel towards any attempt by the official agencies to intervene and control their lives (Little 1990). Craine comments that young people growing up in an area of high unemployment in Manchester were very aware of the respect accorded to those who can afford a lavish life style, and were aware of the criminal means through which it might be gained. At an early stage in their lives they were aware that, in the community in which they were growing up, "crime *does* pay" in terms of status and life style (Craine 1994). Further, Carlen has presented a depressing picture of the well-worn career path from care to custody for young women leaving local authority care (Carlen 1988). She analyses "the complex interplay of class, racism and gender" within this process, showing how these constitute a powerful means through which young women in and leaving care can conceive of little alternative but to engage in criminal behaviour. Of course they had choices other than to engage in crime. And the care system which looked after them so badly had different choices too. But for young people leaving care, the choice is often between the devil and the deep blue sea.

The choice of an illegal "method" depends on the environment in which young people live, the groups with which they associate and the stage of their career development. We have already seen that there are different peak ages of offending for different sorts of crime. In a small-scale intensive study of 45 young men who later became serious and persistent offenders, Little points out that first offences were rarely if ever planned or sophisticated. The examples he cites are driving a stolen car or breaking into a shop where this often was done on the spur of the moment and frequently resulted in either disaster (a crash) or very little tangible reward – goods that were of no use and couldn't be sold (Little 1990). As others confirm, such activities are often part of a subculture of hanging around on the street, "doing nothing", and most likely to be committed as a member of a group or gang of the same age (Corrigan 1976, Foster 1990). In this sense, early youth crime is often spontaneous, unskilled, committed by a peer group having a bit of a laugh together, and acted out as a piece of hooliganism rather than as a piece of calculated or instrumental criminality. In that a lot of it is opportunistic, much will be determined by particular circumstances and be subject to the ebbs and flows of youth subcultural "leisure preoccupations" – hence the prevalence of car- and football-related crime. In his study of young people growing up in inner city Manchester in the 1980s, Craine points out that some of this opportunistic crime was often associated with travelling football supporters, as all part of a good day out, or an exciting foray on to the Continent for a European away match. He reports that during the 1980s travelling supporters developed patterns of "steaming" – a highly direct, unsophisticated, but temporarily successful means of stealing from shops by hordes of supporters who would dash into and through shops grabbing handfuls of seemingly random selections of the goods on display (Craine 1994). As with other forms of ritual football violence in the 1970s reported on by Marsh, among others, this can be, and now is, largely policed out of existence, or at least displaced by police action (Marsh et al. 1978). Particular types of youth crime do, therefore, come and go almost like a fashion as different opportunities arise or are "closed off" by effective policing.

There is a sense in which this "opportunistic and recreational crime" is supported, sustained and legitimated by youth subcultures which do not regard it as in any way "really serious". This is also true of the early involvement of young people in a drug subculture in which drug taking is seen as being just part of, and enhancing, a good night out and is certainly distanced in their minds from the "dangerous drug-taking behaviour" of others. Many of the young adults described by Merchant & MacDonald as taking Ecstasy before raves were candid about its value in enhancing their leisure and careful in taking proper precautions to avoid its worst side-effects (Merchant & MacDonald 1994). Yet in all these "recreational crimes", despite not resulting in any substantial material gain (even when it involves committing burglary, as in Little's study), young people often report on the excitement associated with the first acts of deviance and crime. Although fun, with the benefit of hindsight this is also regarded as being slightly ridiculous (Foster 1990, Little 1990).

These studies also point out that the communities in which such acts occur often regard them as the "natural" behaviour of "boys being boys" (Foster 1990, Little 1990) or fully-fledged ravers doing what ravers do and being both "high and happy" (Merchant & MacDonald 1994). This subcultural setting for early crime is also associated with its *justifications*, the third element of Farrington's model. Many writers make reference to Sykes & Matza's notion of "techniques of neutralisation" through which young people define their deviant acts as harmless and legitimate (Sykes & Matza 1957).

Thus, for contemporary young offenders, TWOC becomes "joy-riding", vandalism is redefined as "having a 'laff' " – a piece of excitement to alleviate boredom – and even theft, harassment and assault are regarded as not intentionally inflicting serious harm or damage on to people who are thought of as being provocative – "asking for it", and not really harmed (Campbell 1993, Corrigan 1976, Craine 1994, Foster 1990, Marsh et al. 1978).

In two separate studies by Foster and Craine we are given rare insights into young people's involvement in crime through the reports of ethnographic field work undertaken in South London and Manchester respectively. Both show how the development of criminality and criminal opportunity structures are deeply rooted in the institutions of the two different local communities. The titles of the two studies are illuminating in that, while Foster's study is called simply *Villains*, Craine makes clear the pragmatics of career choice in calling his *Beggars can't be choosers* (Craine 1994, Foster 1990). Craine describes the way in which the young people in his study regarded their chances of any legitimate employment career as bleak and had respect for older young people who "made out" by being "on the fiddle". He also outlines the strategic role of two market dynasties who offered both semi- and illegitimate employment opportunities to the young searching for ways of making a living. In these forms of "employment", the young people in his study were taught by those around them how to fiddle the benefit system to supplement their wages and offered other forms of other more lucrative and illegal means of earning a living, through "barking", "touting" and "hustling". Getting the few jobs available within the community, therefore, acted both as an apprenticeship in learning other "fiddles" and as access to a social network which could offer other forms of "employment" on the edges of crime, something confirmed by ethnographic work done by MacDonald in the North-East of England (MacDonald 1994). The first of these activities, "barking" (also known elsewhere as "fly-pitching") involved unlicensed street trading. "Touting" involved the sale of both legal and forged tickets for music concerts ("gigs") or sports matches, and "hustling" referred to street-level sales of small amounts of drugs. In the absence of legitimate jobs within the formal labour market, some young people, therefore, availed themselves of these and other semi-legitimate jobs within the informal economy which further gave them access to alter-

187

native "opportunity structures", some of which involved training in the techniques of entrepreneurial crime. What activities such as barking, touting and hustling all had in common were elaborate and developed divisions of labour between members of a group, involving systems of look-outs against apprehension by the police, and lines of supply so that the seller was never in danger of being caught with large quantities of goods at any one time (which might lead to the confiscation of valuable assets as well as constituting a more serious offence). In becoming involved in such activities, young people served an apprenticeship as "dogs" or "dog-outs" before being promoted to the better-paid jobs of being the actual barker, tout or hustler. Foster reports that the one young woman she knew to have been involved in criminal activity had been employed as a dog in a fly-pitching scam for her brother in the market (Foster 1990). Craine also reports that the two market dynasties acted as important means through which more developed and organized crime such as "hoisting" (large-scale shop lifting) was done "to order" and for a fixed price. One group of young people he studied had developed this into a highly elaborate drama and a lucrative business by their late teens and early twenties, one episode of which he was called upon to witness (Craine 1994). Although the local community offered them an easy means through which to fence the goods they stole, they were often willing and able to plan and carry out their activities across wide geographical areas. As they did so, they made good use of the skills they had learnt in their early apprenticeships; working to elaborate divisions of labour, carefully co-ordinated team work, careful timing and, above all, a profound sense of team loyalty. Taylor has indicated that this is a hallmark of older professional criminals (Taylor 1984).

Members of the hoisting gang described by Craine were well established in their careers in crime. Before this stage is attained, as Little also argues, they had gone through several other phases in which their beliefs and activities had moved on from "delinquency as fun". Little points out that the criminal career "is not a smooth journey, it is a series of bumps and starts" (Little 1990: 85). As a young person becomes a more serious and persistent offender, excitement becomes less likely to be the prime motive, though Little claims there is considerable pride in the "bottle" involved. He reports that persistent offenders accept a status as being "outsiders" in the community, more isolated from, or marginal to, mainstream groups (Little 1990). As Craine and others testify, offending is often done as part of a small, tightly controlled group, which acts cohesively, to a carefully orchestrated game plan and with intense loyalty through which it can rescue any member at risk of being caught (Craine 1988, Taylor 1984).

Little's study is a study of "failures" in the sense that all his subjects had been caught and ended up in custody. But he is able to trace the ways in which custody itself gave a further twist to the development of young criminal careers. Initial incarceration is reported as being traumatic and shocking. The number of suicides in prison bears testimony to the fact that some young people simply do not cope with the penalties of failure (Howard League for Penal Reform 1993a). Many young men in Little's study had experienced residential care before being committed to custodial institutions for young offenders. Yet the language they used about youth custody was that of adult prisoners popularized and glamorized by television series such as *Porridge*. The young men describe a bleak life dominated by working the "screws", being "banged up" for long periods of time, "slopping out" and occasional bouts of "exercise" and "association". To survive imprisonment, they learnt the script but also developed considerable self-reliance and a belief in the importance of maintaining a distance from, and a manipulative stance towards, those in authority. He also confirms that these institutions served to increase and broaden their knowledge and skills of how better to commit crime and, as such, acted as a "university of crime" (Little 1990).

Prevention of criminal careers and careers out of crime

This review of the social correlates of persistent offending and the factors involved in the development of criminal careers can help to set a policy agenda for crime prevention. We need to understand properly if we are to intervene effectively. First we have seen that multiple social and economic deprivation during the early years of childhood is a predictor of persistent offending during the years of youth. Similarly, later disinvolvement from education leads to low educational achievement and a greater likelihood of youth crime. Sadly, as we saw in Chapter 6, this is highly likely to occur for young people brought up in the public care. Unsupervised and unstructured youth leisure time and boredom on the streets were reported to be associated with minor acts of delinquency, some of which gave young people the taste for excitement associated with delinquency and criminal activity. The lack of clear opportunity structures into legitimate employment also encourages early dabbling in the informal economy which, as we have seen, may further introduce young people to opportunity structures involving crime and benefit fraud. Living in communities where the visible signs of a successful life style enjoyed by people engaged in crime further acted to entice young people into believing that this was the only real way in which they were going to obtain social status or make a decent living. Some among the young perceive crime to be largely victimless, socially acceptable and worth the small risk of being apprehended. Only among the criminal failures, who were caught and committed to custodial sentences, was there a perception that their future lives were likely to be blighted by early offending. This mainly led them to learn how to be more careful and skilful in offending, instrumental and far-sighted in planning crime, and less trustful of those around them (Little 1990).

This summary suggests that policy intervention can be planned at a number of different phases in the development of young criminal careers. First, we should examine what can be done during the early years of a young person's life so as to prevent disinvolvement from the educational process, and sustain educational motivation through the difficult years of their early teens. Second, we should address patterns of leisure provision for the young and how these can be appropriately and acceptably structured and supervised. Thirdly, we should examine how the techniques of neutralization can be reversed so that young people recognize the serious harm done to the victims of crime, by what many regard as harmless pranks. This can also involve greater consideration of what can be done to make offenders face the long-term life-course consequences of persistent criminal behaviour. Fourthly, we must also address what can be done to help those who are caught committing crimes to cease their offending behaviour at an early stage in its development. Given that most minor offenders will remain within the community rather than be consigned to custody, we must address what can be done within the community. Finally, we must ask what can be done for those who do receive custodial offences to prepare them for legitimate careers once they are released.

190

As we have seen, poor performance during the early years of schooling, truanting and low levels of educational qualification are all associated with later persistent offending. One obvious strategy to reduce later offending is, therefore, to try to ensure that those most likely to be educationally disadvantaged and those who reject education receive what in the United States is called a "head start". While this is obviously a *long-term* measure, with a time lag in terms of its effectiveness in preventing crime of ten or more years, experience in the United States suggests that such investment can bring enormous dividends. The "Perry Pre-School Programme" involved a comparison of the fortunes of two groups of disadvantaged black children brought up in the town of Ypsilanti in the State of Michigan. One group of children was given early nursery schooling between the ages of 3 and 5, while another, matched, control group was not. By the early 1990s the groups had reached the age of 27. A report on the scheme produced in 1993 claims that those who had been given nursery education were more likely to have finished high school, more likely to have higher levels of literacy, and more likely to have obtained better jobs. They would, furthermore, be less likely to have needed the intervention of social services, and less likely to have grown up to be persistent offenders. By the age of 27, only 7% of the experimental group had been arrested five or more times compared with 35% of the control group (Schweinhart & Weikhart 1993). The report estimates that, for every $1 million dollars invested in the programme, the state had saved $7 million in reduced expenditure on special education, lost tax revenue and costs incurred through the criminal justice system. This is powerful evidence that investment in crime prevention must take a long-term perspective and address the wide range of welfare needs of potential offenders (Utting et al. 1993).

The "Perry Pre-School Programme" also involved home visits to attempt to replicate "child-initiated" structured activity within the school with similar activities at home. In reviewing good pre-school education in Britain, Woodhead has argued that it can "engender, re-enforce and sustain parental aspirations and interests in their child's education [and so promote] long term educational and social competence" (Woodhead, quoted by Utting et al. 1993: 46). In the United Kingdom, only 13% of mothers of children who had attended local authority nursery provision had been involved in activities in the nursery in any way (Utting et al. 1993). A similar programme to that developed in the United States is currently being piloted in four "demonstration projects" in Lewisham, Liverpool, Manchester and Newcastle and funded by the Home Office, although, perhaps disappointingly, the important school–family links are not being replicated. It deserves wider application. Failure to spend on nursery education now is likely to cost dearly on the budgets of welfare services at a later date. The success of the US programme goes some way to explaining why all main British political parties are now committed to nursery education as a welfare priority for the mid-1990s.

The second phase of intervention we identified concerned the leisure activities of young people in their early teens. The most obvious form of provision which might address this issue is, of course, the youth service. Yet the development of much youth work in the United Kingdom has been associated with the education service and is often located in schools or youth annexes attached to schools (Davies 1986, Jeffs & Smith 1988). To those already disenchanted with school, this physical identification with school does not enhance the attractiveness of such provision. Furthermore, as a non-statutory arm of the education service, the youth service has suffered cuts in funding at precisely the time that it is most needed. There is therefore an urgent need to review leisure provision for young people. The 1970s saw the development of detached youth workers who were encouraged to make contact with young people wherever they were to be found. Yet, unlike similar schemes in other parts of the world, these workers have been dependent upon their own wits and skills and receive little or no specialized training for their work (Chow 1992). This is another area of policy and provision which requires urgent attention.

A number of pilot projects have addressed the need to resensitize young people to the effects of crime on the lives of their victims and on their own future prospects. This is the third phase we identified as important if we are to reverse the "techniques of neutralization" which act as a mental buffer between offenders and the consequences of their actions. Yet projects designed to address these issues have received only precarious funding. The "Anti-Crime Encounter Initiative" run by the Probation Service in Merseyside and the Mersey Care Trust employed an ex-serious offender to talk to schoolchildren, emphasizing the effects of crime on victims and the harrowing and debilitating effects of prison. Yet the Home Office has refused to continue the funding of this project (*Independent* 20 October 1993).

The vast majority of young offenders are dealt with by the police or courts through either administering cautions or through Community or Probation Orders. In the late 1980s the National Association for the Care and Resettlement of Offenders (NACRO) illustrated that projects to divert young people from crime and treat offenders within the community can be successful (NACRO 1991b). Even those who may later be given a custodial sentence will, before their appearance in court, be in the community on bail and there is considerable concern for young people who commit crime while on bail (House of Commons 1993). The fourth phase at which we need to direct policy better is the support of young offenders in the community. A number of imaginative schemes have been developed to support offenders, to help steer them away from crime, and to displace the widespread incidence of car-related crime through "motor projects". Following a survey of all local authorities, conducted in the spring of 1993, NACRO reported that in a third of all areas, there is no bail support scheme nor arrangements for support for those who have been cautioned. "Motor projects" for young offenders existed in only half of the areas covered by the survey, and only one-third had any remand fostering arrangement in place (NACRO 1993). While most local authorities were of the opinion that even persistent offenders were capable of being "managed" within the community, only 28 of the 110 authorities covered by the survey considered that the level of provision they had made was adequate to meet needs. NACRO calls for both guidance and ring-fenced additional funding for local authorities to develop services which are of critical importance in preventing the drift into serious crime or persistent offending. Without it, crime is likely to continue at an immense cost to the tax payer. The 1993 Select Committee report called for attention to be paid to cost-effective means of reducing juvenile crime when estimates were drawn up for the allocation of local authority grants from central government (House of Commons 1993).

The fifth area of concern is the treatment of young offenders within custody. We have already pointed out that custody can enhance a young person's criminal knowledge and skills. Yet time in custody can also be a time during which educational and vocational skills and qualifications are acquired. Where this is provided in Local Authority

Community Homes and Youth Treatment Centres this can be seen to reduce later offending (Bullock et al. 1994a, Ditchfield & Catan 1992). Yet the education service within prisons is under threat and due to be privatized. Training schemes and Job Clubs specially designed for ex-offenders and run by those with specialist knowledge, such as NACRO, have been allowed to wither because they were deemed more expensive than non-specialist schemes. And as we have seen, innovative programmes such as the Nightingale scheme in Feltham YOI depend upon untrained staff and private charity. There is an urgent need to review not only the level and type of education and training provision in custodial institutions, but also the training of staff and their potential in arranging systems of "throughcare".

Finally, we must draw attention to the important economic context of criminal behaviour and recidivism. The relationship between (un)employment and crime is complex (Coles & Fowles 1991, Crow 1989). Yet Crow calculated that a 1 per cent rise in unemployment was correlated with 163 young people being received into custody, which in effect adds more than £1 million pounds to the Home Office budget. Just as investment in pre-school education can be shown to be a cost-effective means of preventing persistent offending in later life, so we can not expect the pursuit of a career in crime to be diverted without an expansion of opportunity structures for legitimate careers in the labour market.

"Happily ever after"?

Gaining good education and training and a legitimate job are not the only aspirations of young people. These are only one dimension of the youth transitions we identified in Chapter 1. Setting up partnerships and leaving home are also important elements in the process of becoming adult citizens. The hoisting gangs studied by Craine were well established in their careers and saw little future in "straight" and legal means of earning a living. It is perhaps significant that few of them were involved in stable partnerships with members of the opposite sex. Yet a number of studies have pointed out that while large numbers of young people are involved in (often petty) crime, this ceases as they reach their late teens and early 20s. Foster points to the influence of the significant role women play in policing the behaviour of young men (Foster 1990). Girlfriends are reported as the main group responsible for enticing young men off the streets and out of offending. She reports that during their late teens young men and women spend considerable amounts of time in each other's company, indeed she regards this as a unique time in the life cycle in which men and women are together for longer periods of time than at any other time of their lives. Like other studies, she points to the ways in which young women attempt to make certain that their boyfriends do not indulge in (too much) risk-taking behaviour or actions which could put their relationship at risk were young men to be arrested, convicted and sent to prison. The behaviour of the late-teenage young men she studied indicates that they were more calculating in terms of assessing risk and realized that persistent offending might jeopardize their legitimate activity as drivers, workers and partners. Jenkins, in a study of a similar age group of young working-class men on the outskirts of Belfast, and Coffield et al. in a study in the North-East, both report a similar civilizing influence of girlfriends (Coffield et al. 1986, Jenkins 1983). Yet, the lack of legitimate employment opportunities for young men has been argued to make them seem a less than attractive proposition to young women (Wallace 1987). Some have argued that it reduces the "marriageable pool" of young men, and freezes them outside citizenship in the depths of the young "underclass" (Halsey 1993). If we are to be serious in our attempt to address both crime and the causes of crime, we must address all these issues in a coherent and holistic approach to all the dimensions of youth transitions.

Chapter Nine

Beyond the underclass debate and towards a framework for youth policy into the twenty-first century

This book has reviewed our understanding of youth, the ways in which the transitions of youth have been affected by recent social and economic changes in Britain, and the legal and social policy context in which young people's welfare is determined. We have employed two major concepts to aid our understanding of these issues. First, we have described youth transitions in terms of *career* – status sequences through which young people pass between childhood and adulthood. The use of this concept enables us to examine the ways in which the major transitions of youth are shaped both by the structures of opportunity open to young people, and the decisions they, and others around them, make as they move from one status to another. It has been argued that it is particularly important for social policy to concentrate attention upon career rather than trajectory. This is not to deny the profound influence of social and economic forces in shaping the life chances of young people – indeed, much of this book has outlined their fundamental importance. To concentrate attention on career, however, does offer an insight into areas of policy development which might change decision-making processes of both young people and those around them and thereby potentially change career outcomes.

Secondly, we have employed the concept of *citizenship* and refined our understanding of this term to unpack a complex of needs, rights and interests which young people might claim to have. Meeting these claims to citizenship involves including young people within the community as full participant members, ensuring that they are not exploited or abused and that their welfare is sustained and supported. As we have examined young people's careers in the 1990s, however, it is clear that many of them are being excluded from full citizenship, have their needs unmet, have their rights ignored, and have their interests vetoed by the interests of others.

Despite the wishes of the Prime Minister in his speech made upon his general election victory in 1992, Britain is not a classless society. This book has outlined a number of structures of disadvantage which stratify youth transitions. Previous studies of youth have focused attention on the divisions of social class, gender, ethnicity and region, all of which offer young people differentiated structures of opportunity (Banks et al. 1992, Bates & Riseborough 1993, Jones & Wallace 1992). This book has attempted to highlight three further dimensions of difference and disadvantage: being brought up in the public care; having a disability or special need; involvement in crime and the criminal justice system. In Chapter 1 we described the transitions as akin to an elaborate game of snakes and ladders. As the changing nature of youth transitions has been examined, we have seen how many transitions are extended by social and economic change. Most young people still manage to scramble up the (albeit extended) ladders of transition to adulthood and citizenship. But many do not. We have also, therefore, described a number of fractured transitions and the circumstances in which these are most likely to occur. As disadvantaged young people slip down the snakes of further disadvantage and exclusion, they are left unemployed, homeless, isolated, excluded from mainstream society and marginalized from the means through which they can enhance their future welfare.

In designing better social policies for young people, we must be concerned to ensure that the ladders of opportunity are more secure and the routes to them properly signposted, so that all involved in the promotion of the welfare careers of young people can help to guarantee that wise and beneficial decisions are taken, and that these are made at the right time. But social policies must also be cognizant about, and concerned for, those young people who lose their way. Policy must, therefore, address the needs of the young unemployed, the homeless and the isolated, as well as protecting young people from exploitation, harassment or abuse as they attempt the youth transitions. Failed and fractured transitions are sometimes highly visible. It has become commonplace in the 1990s to see signs of home-

197

lessness, unemployment and destitution, as well as to experience private property crime and disorder in public places, both committed predominantly by the young. There is also widespread public concern about teenage pregnancy, drug abuse and begging. But it should be remembered that, throughout history, young people have been associated with "trouble" (Pearson 1983). As Hebdige argues, young people pose, pose as threat, and pose a threat to the community and social order. Yet when they do so, they often get talked about, listened to, and their grievances acted upon. He further points out that while troublesome youth get arrested, admonished, disciplined and incarcerated, they are also often emulated (Hebdige 1988). Troublesome youth can be fashionable as well as the subject of public concern and moral panics (Cohen 1980). This too has always been the case. Yet some would have us believe that we are in a new dark age and that what has emerged with the growing number of fractured youth transitions is a new and dangerous underclass of predatory young people for whom there is no way back to civilized society and citizenship.

New times and the growth of a youth underclass?

In reviewing youth transitions within the pages of this book, there are times when the attraction of the concept of the underclass may have seemed apparent. As we reviewed changes in the labour market in Chapter 2 it became clear that young people were more likely than older groups to experience unemployment, and that those who became dis-involved in education and who did worst at school were the most likely to be unemployed. In reviewing changing family structures in Chapter 3, it was apparent that there has been a growth in single and lone parenthood, as well as a growth in the numbers of young people living in reconstituted families. Furthermore, there is some evidence that young people brought up in these conditions experience disadvantages. We reported evidence suggesting that it is those young people who are most likely to have experienced disrupted home lives and educational disadvantages, who attempt early transitions to the labour market, independent living and family formations. Those who left home "prematurely" were, furthermore, most likely to experience unemployment and homelessness (Jones 1993a). As we reviewed young people's involvement in crime in the last chapter, it was also clear that, where young people grow up in circumstances where the traditional transitions offer few legitimate opportunities, other illegitimate opportunity structures are likely to develop and many young people will avail themselves of these.

If unemployment, family breakdown, low educational achievement and criminality are connected, do we not need to be able to conceptualize and theorize the relationships between these to understand properly the new times in which we live? Does this apparent interconnectedness add up to mounting evidence of a youth underclass? Morris has indicated that underclass is often used to conjure up images of the perishing and dangerous classes, a "mischievous ambiguity" of the deserving and undeserving poor, and is sometime used as a means of apportioning moral blame on the victims of social and economic exclusion (Morris 1994). Campbell has also pointed out that the term "underclass" also carries a spatial connotation. It is clear that some of the greatest disadvantages are to be found in working-class council estates, which she evocatively describes as "the edge of a class and the end of the city" (Campbell 1993: 319). The estate has become a symbol of all the symptoms of the underclass. Yet as Campbell also points out, estates are deeply gendered, with the lads on the streets and the lasses in the home. One of the estates on which she reports is the Meadowell Estate in Newcastle which was subjected to rioting in 1991. Dennis too visited this estate, yet he chose to focus on what he regards as the consequences of families without fathers (Dennis & Erdos 1992). Campbell described the gallant attempt of women to win back their communities, to defend their "homes", and to re-create a shared and collective welfare of family and community life in spaces synonymous with male crime. Not for her the vague laments or rantings of disillusioned old socialists who see the moral fabric of society threatened by such pernicious effects of women's liberation as Prudential advertisements ridiculing stay-at-home males (Dennis & Erdos 1992). In a bizarre, if sad, foray into the underclass debate, Dennis & Erdos reviewed "the evidence" of the growth of the underclass in Britain. Much of the evidence relating to young people is also reviewed within the pages of this book. But in a footnote to the preface of their book *Families without fatherhood* Dennis & Erdos see fit to quote as evidence the dialogue of an advertisement between a (dumb) male and (career-ambitious) female concerning the relative merits of enjoying the garden (male preference). (There are much better, and more provocative, advertisements in the series now in which the stay-at-home-male wants a baby. She . . . doesn't!) For Dennis & Erdos, it seems, women's liberation provides evidence not only of the lamentable state of gardens on the Meadowell Estate, but of the moral undermining of fatherhood and patriarchally controlled families. Yet is there real evidence of the crucial importance of fathers in controlling the young? As was seen in Chapter 3, it is mothers who both care *and* control even within two-parent families. To seek a solution to the breakdown of law and order in the policing of men back into authority figures within traditional families, as Dennis & Erdos seem to suggest, is to conflate an understanding of family relationships with the castigation of particular types of household structure. Single mothers and lone parents do not cause the breakdown of law and order, the evidence suggests that it is predominantly young men who do. And as we saw in Chapter 8 they are most likely to do so where there are no legitimate opportunity structures for them to get the jobs, houses and stable relationships which the evidence consistently indicates most of them still want (Banks & Ullah 1988). There are, therefore, dangers in displacing a concern for the effects of structural changes in the economy and society into a blame for the private moral commitments parents display for the victims of these changes.

This leads us to an even more serious complaint about underclass theory. Bagguley & Mann provide the clue to the issue in the playful reference to the unemployed, the products of single-parent families, and the criminals as "idle, thieving bastards" (Bagguley & Mann 1992). To be sure, many young people are unemployed, some were born into and were brought up in single-parent families, and some may be guilty of property crime. But, as this book has indicated, many of the young people who are most disadvantaged in attempting youth transitions are difficult to castigate simply with Bagguley & Mann's ironic phrase. Many of the most disadvantaged have been brought up in the public care and yet more are educated in schools dealing with young people with disabilities or special needs. These young people are, therefore, the products of public welfare provision and the sons and daughters of the state in *loci parentis*. Are these the people we would also wish to condemn and castigate with the label "underclass"? Are these young people, whom we do so little to help, to be lumped all together and with those who posed and postured in the riotous escapades described by Campbell? Are there not real political dangers in conceptually lumping together those who may wilfully avoid work and indulge in crime with those not afforded the possibility of work through systems of social discrimination and structural disadvantage? Are we so desperate for catchy labels for the complex malaise in welfare provision that we should embrace the term "underclass" which now carries with it so much ideological baggage? It is worth remembering that the term has been appropriated by the New Right from an author who was concerned for the casualties of structural change in America. For Myrdal, who reintroduced the term "underclass" to our contemporary condition, was most concerned with the impact of economic and structural change on people most vulnerable to its effect (Myrdal 1962). Murray seems much less charitable. He calls, not for more money to be spent on the welfare of the vulnerable, but for the withdrawal of government from what he regards as the failed attempts at social engineering. In Murray's view, communities should be allowed to govern themselves. In one of the most callous sentences in his twisted "thesis" he argues that the social life and problems of others "needn't bother the rest of us too much as long as it stays in its own part of town" (Murray 1990: 35). Can we afford to leave the vulnerable to stew in their own juice? Campbell described the ways in which, as women attempted to win back and control their communities, they were constantly thwarted by both the lack of support from official agencies and their vulnerability to further crime and victimization if they helped to identify the perpetrators of crime and disorder. If communities are to help in constructing and defending the welfare of their members, they also need help and support in doing so. If young people are to lead lives which do not involve acts of crime and disorder, the welfare environment in which they grow up must be one which promotes opportunities for employment, the re-creation of safe and secure families, and active and responsible citizenship in communities to which young people can feel proud to belong. Rather than aiding our understanding of the fractured transitions of youth, underclass theory is, as Walker has argued, "at best, misleading and, at worst, a dangerous diversion from the major problems and deprivations facing Britain" (Murray 1990: 50).

A framework for youth policy and a Ministry for Youth

Underclass theory, therefore, offers no real policy agenda apart from a castigation of the vulnerable and a legitimization of inactivity on the part of government. Yet, if we are to have a more positive policy agenda for young people we must be clear about what the policy objectives are and how they might be best and most effectively pursued. Chapter 4 argued that a distinctive set of welfare needs, rights and interests could be identified which related to the three main transitions of youth: from education to the labour market; from living with the families to attaining some measure of welfare independence from them; from living with families to leaving home and living independently. It was argued, in Chapters 4 and 5, that welfare rights could be usefully subdivided into entitlements, rights of protection, representational rights and enabling rights. The Appendix attempts to develop and summarize these. In outlining an agenda for youth policy it is important to examine which aspects of these rights, needs and interests can be appropriately developed in addressing the three main transitions.

In Chapter 1 we argued that many of the tragedies of youth policy lay in the lack of co-ordination between the different arms and agencies of the state. Chapters 6 and 7 further illustrated this point, as we examined the welfare careers of young people in and leaving the public care and young people with disabilities or special needs. While there has been some legislative change which is attempting to address the most glaring failures of policy co-ordination, recent reviews of the implementation of the Children Act 1989 and the Community Care Act 1990 suggest that there is some considerable way to go if the bold aims of these acts are to be turned into reality (Department of Health 1993). We argue here that there is a continuing need to monitor progress, to assess the youth welfare implications of policy development in separate agencies of the state, and to suggest means through which the youth policy agenda can be further developed and refined. Following Coleman & Warren-Adamson, this book calls for the establishment of a Ministry for Youth (Coleman & Warren-Adamson 1992).

What would such a ministry do and what are the dangers inherent in such a development? Coleman & Warren-Adamson suggest that it might develop "youth impact statements at a national and local level ... seek to provide information and argument for those seeking to plan policy ... [and an] ... interagency perspective" (Coleman & Warren-Adamson 1992). It is clear from these suggestions that the role would be one of co-ordination and of researching and assessing the impact on young people's welfare of other large and powerful ministries of state. It is not envisaged that a Ministry for Youth would be an executive agency but rather that it would oversee the development of a more holistic and co-ordinated approach to policy development and may also provide a vehicle through which non-governmental agencies dealing with young people (and including young people themselves) might share in the development of youth policy.

There are some dangers in having a Ministry for Youth. A research and policy co-ordination and development agency may become merely a talking shop. It may be an irritant to, but marginalized from, the real business of policy implementation by the major departments of state. Furthermore, it may become a token of concern for policy co-ordination, without any real means through which to achieve policy coherence. Yet, in the absence of any attempt to develop a coherent youth policy, serious and damaging differences of direction and emphasis in government policy have developed. It is young people who have suffered the consequences, together with their families and the communities in which they live.

Education, training and the labour market and the transition from school to work

In reviewing Murray's diagnosis of the underclass, both Walker and Deakin argue that the root cause of many of the problems lies in unemployment (Murray 1990). We reviewed the impact of unemployment and the consequent restructuring of the youth labour market in Chapter 2. In all parts of the European Union there is a growing belief that we must face the challenge of creating jobs and regulating a labour market, if obtaining employment is to be a real possibility for all citizens, including the young. There are signs in Britain, for the first time in more than a decade and a half, that significant reductions in the levels of unemployment lie at the top of the political agenda of all the main political parties. How can this concern be turned into policies which will result in more and better job opportunities for young people?

First, we must ensure that young people are well educated and well trained and have the skills employers want. In this sense, education and training policy must be co-ordinated. Chapter 2 also pointed to the growing number of young people who now stay on in education beyond minimum school-leaving age, in the belief that further education will help them gain entry to better-paid and more fulfilling work. Yet, it also pointed to some considerable concern that many young people did so with only the vague hope that they were making the right career decisions and, in a worrying number of cases, poor or ill-advised choices resulted in later failure and drop-out from post-16 courses (Audit Commission–OFSTED 1993). We argued in Chapter 2 that this suggested a need for careful, well-informed, and effective careers guidance and advice for young people faced by difficult choices. There is some evidence that careers education comes too little and too late, is not perceived as helpful by many of the young, lamentably excludes the most strategically important people (parents) from the process, and is too focused on 16-year-olds (Coles 1993). As we reviewed the careers of young people in care and young people with special needs or disabilities in Chapters 7 and 8, it was clear that there was a special and urgent need for proper and effective careers guidance to be given to these groups. As outlined in Chapter 4, these needs are clearly identified within the European Charter on Rights, and some means through which these can be met are envisaged under the Social Chapter for the Maastricht Treaty. Britain's opt-out from the Social Chapter must not mean that these needs are not adequately addressed.

Secondly, as was argued in Chapter 7, opportunities for education, training and work are of critical importance to *all* young people, including those with special needs or disabilities. In previous decades many young people with disabilities, who are now excluded from the labour market, did secure work. When they are unemployed, they are just as likely to suffer the social and psychological damage caused by unemployment as occurs to others (Banks & Ullah 1988). When young people with disabilities do get a job this can make a dramatic difference to their social skills, their feelings of self-worth, their general welfare, as well as providing them with an important source of income. Chapter 7 made clear, however, that not all young people with severe disabilities will be able to obtain open employment. But we argued that young people with a disability or special needs should have a right to packages of care which included education, training, work and social security, as well as health and social support. We further argued that, while partnerships between private employers and voluntary groups working with the disabled are to be encouraged, the rights of those with disabilities not to be discriminated against must be made clear by an act of Parliament.

Thirdly, in attempting to secure rights to appropriate education, training and careers education and guidance we must not ignore rights *at work* and *in training*. Young workers are often inexperienced, unaware of their employment rights, and are rarely consulted about their rates of pay or the conditions under which they work. They are sometimes also subject to abuse and harassment at work and in circumstances in which they feel there is little or nothing they can do except tolerate this or leave and become unemployed. The rights of young people at work and in training do, therefore, clearly need to be specially protected. This applies to those working full time and those engaged in part-time work while continuing their education. In Chapter 2 we drew attention to the ways in which the law on children working was widely disregarded, with many being employed under age, during hours prohibited by law, and sometimes in conditions which jeopardized both their health and safety and their educational development. Given the expansion of this sector of the economy, it is important that part-time work is subject to monitoring and regulation. The present system for this is clearly not working and urgently needs to be reviewed. The government's commitment to labour market flexibility and its stand against regulation from Europe has, for the moment, excluded many areas of young people's rights at work from any form of regulation. Should we adopt the Social Chapter of the *Maastricht Treaty* in the future, this will be one means through which the special rights of young people at work can be signalled. This will also include their representational rights to consultation in the workplace. There is, however, also a need to examine in more detail how the implementation of these rights can be properly monitored and fulfilled.

Fourthly, if we have to assume that some young people will be unemployed at some time in their careers, we must urgently rethink their entitlement to benefit, the conditions under which such entitlements will be met and what might be expected of them while they remain economically inactive. One of the more difficult issues to be faced is balancing the need to provide young people with the means of not being exploited while in training or work, destitute or suffering welfare harm when unemployed or on poorly paid training schemes, without making the benefits paid while unemployed outweigh the advantages of working or training. Various forms of community service are currently being suggested (*Independent* 31 May 1994). While these may offer opportunities for young people to contribute to the community and thus genuinely enhance active youth citizenship, the dangers with any new schemes are that they will be regarded with suspicion by the young. In the 1990s, the latter have lived a lifetime which has seen so many attempts at repackaging training and schemes under different brand names and it will be difficult to convince many of them that, this time, it is different. The key may be to offer remuneration which is commensurate with the value of the work being undertaken.

Social care and social protection

The social policy agenda for young people must, therefore, do much more than provide a healthy economic context for free labour markets to operate, the protection of young people at work, and the social protection of those who are unemployed. The pathways to successful youth transitions lie far back in childhood. In Chapter 8 we reviewed evidence from the United States about the long-term benefits of investing in nursery education and family support, and the long-term consequences of allowing disinvolvement from, or underperformance in, the education system. In Chapter 6 we reviewed evidence which suggested that the failure of the state in adequately promoting the welfare of young people who are brought up in care left these young people among the most disadvantaged and the most vulnerable sections of the community. Means must be found to secure the bold aims of the Children Act 1989, that young people in care must be given extra help with their education rather than less, extra support from all around them in their choices of career at the age of 16, and rights of consultation and regimes of care which will serve to empower rather than diminish them. This is a bold agenda and a severe task for those charged with meeting these objectives. Only when these are met, and the system is adequately resourced, will young people in care be able to plan adequately and effectively for their own futures, rather than stumble from care carrying the burdens of abuse, disadvantage and blighted ambitions.

The regulation of the housing market for young people

In Chapter 3 we reviewed the concept of housing career and indicated that for most young people this is rarely a simple, one-step, or unilinear process. As we indicated, many young people leave the parental home but frequently return to it, sometimes because their early attempts at independent living have proved disastrous and resulted in either homelessness or huge debts they could not service. Many people initially leave home to study or to gain employment. And while many colleges and universities provide accommodation for their students in colleges and on campuses with social support services, many others have to live in private rented accommodation.

Jones has reviewed a number of changes in housing provision and the regulation of the housing market and the assumptions on which government policy towards youth homelessness seem to be based (Jones 1993a). She has suggested that, when young people do not meet the assumptions government makes about living at home; being dependent upon parents during the transition to independent living, and not leaving until it is economically viable to do so, they run great risks of becoming homeless. Yet, even where young people leave home to get a job (one of the more traditional reasons for leaving), they face real problems in securing accommodation in an increasingly deregulated housing market. Leaving home and being geographically mobile is often the only way in which young people can realistically seek work when they live in communities where local labour markets have collapsed. Yet, in Britain, the housing stock is not designed for geographically mobile, young and single people. In Chapter 3 we reviewed the foyers system based upon a nation-wide system of supported hostel accommodation in France. In many superficial ways this seems to provide an obvious answer to the housing needs of young people moving away from the parental home. If universities provide accommodation in a supportive community for those who benefit from higher education, is not a similar system of welfare care for others equally appropriate? If campus accommodation built in the 1960s is good enough for the sons and daughters of the predominantly middle classes, is not similar provision for *all* young people in the 1990s equally desirable? Yet the introduction of foyers to Britain has received a mixed response (Baldwin 1994, Chatrik 1994a, Quilgars & Anderson 1993). Reviewing this in Chapter 3, we again had to point to the lack of policy co-ordination between different arms of the state as the structure of benefits seemed to offer disincentives for young people to break the no home, no job cycle by undertaking training while availing themselves of hostel accommodation. And, in the same way as training in Britain has become associated in the minds of the young with an exploitative response to unemployment, the provision of training hostels runs the risk of being seen as a "homelessness measure" rather than as a positive means of addressing the housing needs of young people in a society in which geographical mobility is often required. Clearly, there are no single solutions to the housing needs of young people. But foyers, where properly developed and run, offer an opportunity where the distinctive housing needs of young people might be met. If they are to be successful they must be developed in ways which safeguard the rights of young people to a modicum of care, support and welfare, while not treating them as problems to be remedied by the paternalistic hand of welfare specialists. Foyers need to become resources which young people can develop and use, not repositories into which social problems can be deposited and controlled out of the way of those who, like the Prime Minister Mr Major, shrink from the welfare needs of homeless beggars.

Investing in the future

This book has reviewed a range of social policy areas affecting youth transitions. In this chapter we have suggested a number of areas where we need to think carefully in developing an agenda for youth policy in the remainder of this decade and into the next century. In the Appendix we provide a checklist of young people's rights which have been distilled from the arguments advanced in the chapters of the book. It has become an aphorism of both academics and politicians that, in investing in young people – through education, training or welfare provision – we are investing in the next generation of citizens. We have outlined the costs of policy failure in terms of wasted lives, missed opportunities and blighted careers. The policy agenda which has been developed will involve considerable public investment, none of which has been costed in this book. It is the firm conviction of the author that it is high time we balance an understandable concern for the cost of investing in youth policy with a recognition of the huge cost of policy failures in terms of the financial burdens to both the state and families of unemployment, homelessness and youth crime. This chapter has condemned those who wish to turn a blind eye to the problems of the vulnerable and leave them alone to their own devices well away from the gaze of public scrutiny. Young people do face problems in developing their own welfare careers. It is in all of our interests that they do so successfully. We can no longer afford to let them fail.

Towards a paradigm of rights for young people

It has been argued in this book that, in developing young people's rights, it is useful to concentrate upon those which affect the three major transitions of youth: from school to work; from family of origin to family of destination; from living with families or surrogate families to living independently. Chapter 4 identified four different sorts of rights: *entitlements* (or legal and moral rights) – the rights to have, do, or know something; *protection rights* – through which young people can be protected from exploitation and abuse; *representational rights* – rights to be involved in decision making, and to be helped and supported in the processes of decision making; and finally *enabling rights*, including rights to the resources, – to help to translate formal rights into real opportunities. Below we codify these further into a set of rights designed to enhance the welfare of youth transitions grouped under the four basic headings.

A. Rights and entitlements

(i) First, young people should be regarded as having:
– **rights to knowledge**
This has particular importance in the fulfilment of their educational needs. Some knowledge claims may be made on the grounds of what, in Chapter 4, was described as "self-actualization" – a claim that citizens should be given the means through which they can be responsible for their own futures (Doyal & Gough 1992). In this sense, we

need knowledge and skills in order to participate in adult society, including the labour market and the political institutions of civil society.

Rights to knowledge can be broken down into the different types of knowledge required of the full citizen. At its most basic:
- **young people need knowledge about their rights.**

Without knowledge about what these are, there is little chance that young people will attempt to fulfil them and, correspondingly, a likelihood that others will abuse them. Of particular importance here is that we can clearly identify rights to knowledge affecting the three main transitions and the three dimensions of disadvantage identified in the first chapter. This means that the following must be included within rights to knowledge:
- **rights to education;**
- **rights to vocational training** of all young people including those with disabilities (as laid down in the European Charter of Rights);
- **rights to knowledge about housing provision including Housing Benefits;**
- **rights to knowledge about Income Support and other forms of social security entitlement**
- **rights to knowledge about health care and health promotion** (including access to knowledge about substance abuse, contraception and abortion);
- **rights to knowledge about the law and the operation of the criminal justice system;**
- **rights to knowledge about entitlements while in care and rights on leaving care.**

(ii) Secondly, young people should be regarded as having:
- **rights to social care, including the right not to be homeless, and rights to social security.**

As has been outlined in Chapter 5, some elements of the above are present in the Children Act 1989. As was also indicated in Chapters 2, and 5, there has been considerable erosion of some of these rights through the withdrawal of Income Support and Housing Benefit. Given what is known about the social composition of the homeless, there is an urgent need for these rights to social care to be diligently and dispassionately assessed. Government policy has acted on the *assumption* that the social care of young people *should be, and is,* primarily provided for within the family. Critics of government policy have provided considerable evidence that, for a large number of young people, *empirically* this is not so. If these rights are to mean anything, we must make certain that there are adequate procedures to ensure that the right to social care is *actually* being met for *all* young people.

(iii) Our discussion of the Children Act 1989 indicated that there is some recognition of:
 – the rights to privacy of young people.
Yet, if this is a right to which young people in care can lay claim, we must argue that it must be considered as a basic welfare right of *all* and should be used as a benchmark for the assessment of conditions under which all young people live.

(iv) Again with respect to the Children Act 1989, we drew attention to:
 – rights to knowledge and respect for cultural and ethnic origins.
As was argued in Chapter 6, while this is now accepted to be of particular importance in dealing with young people in care, it must be asserted as a right of *all* young people and in *all* circumstances.

(v) We now turn to a claim for:
 – rights to equal opportunities.
An abundance of evidence reviewed within this book, and elsewhere, defines the transitions of youth as means through which the social and economic inequalities of the parent generation are reproduced as differential life chances for children and young people (Banks et al. 1992, Bates & Riseborough 1993, Jones & Wallace 1992). Much of the concern has been translated into programmes of education and systems of monitoring service delivery, designed to prevent discrimination on the grounds of class, gender, ethnicity and locality, and to strive for a welfare environment which encourages all to achieve to the best of their ability (see, for instance, Arnot & Weiner 1987, Coles & Maynard 1990, Cross et al. 1990). In Chapter 1 and Part 2 of this book, attention has been directed to the special needs of other groups: young people in care; young people with disabilities; young people with special educational needs; young people in custody. Discussion of these groups makes it clear that ensuring *equal opportu-*

nity does not mean granting the same access to rights and resources.
The discussion of the Children Act 1989, in particular, made it clear
that there must be:
  – a right to *compensatory* care,
if anything approaching real equality of opportunities is to be attained. It has been further argued that any rights granted to young
people can be undermined by the material inequalities of their parents. It is, therefore, important that rights to *compensatory* care be
borne in mind when considering the implementation of the rights of
all young people.

(vi) Rights to care must be dependent upon need. For those with special needs and disabilities we claim a range of rights to ensure that
their needs are properly assessed and identified; that they are properly consulted in this; and that they are given adequate packages of
education training and care from identified sources.
  For young people with special needs and disabilities we claim
  the:
  – right to the assessment of need in education, training, employ-
    ment, health, housing, and social care;
  – right of consultation in the assessment of need;
  – right of appeal against the assessment of need;
  – right to advocacy independent of service providers (if re-
    quested);
  – right to vocational guidance, advice and training;
  – right of regular access to some form of structured social activity;
  – right to health protection and health promotion;
  – right to social security commensurate with special needs;
  – right to have a clear and written explanation of these rights;
  – right to have a named person in an identified service as respon-
    sible for the provision of these services.

(vii) We have mentioned that all young people should be regarded as
having:
  – rights to knowledge which must include knowledge about
    health matters (and, thus, knowledge about sexuality, the conse-
    quences of sexual behaviours, drug use and abuse and the conse-
    quences of risk-taking behaviour).
The Children Act 1989 made clear that for young people over the age

of 16 a claim for knowledge about health matters should also include:
- **rights over their own bodies** (in the sense of being able to seek treatment without the intervention of other people and especially parents or legal guardians).

This must further include:
- **the right to consent to treatment without being over-ruled by others.**

The legal position of young people under the age of 16 was seen to be made more problematic by the Children Act 1989, in that the "autonomy" of a young person's decision is to be adjudicated by doctors. Even so, legally, doctors are to adjudicate under a guiding principle which depends upon the perceived ability of a young person to understand, and maturely reflect upon, the nature of the health condition or illness about which they are being consulted. This right over their own body, is, therefore, argued to be a conditional right for young people under the age of consent.

(viii) The inquiry into "pindown" regimes, used to control young people in care, indicates that serious welfare harm can result from regimes which impose social and emotional, as well as material, restrictions on young people. This makes clear that young people should be granted:
- **rights of association with other young people**

in order to foster their proper social and emotional development. This right, we argue, must be generalizable to *all* young people. The above catalogue of rights has considerable implications for the treatment of young people in a number of different social institutions.

B. Rights of protection

Much of the recent concern with the protection rights of young people has focused on sexual and physical abuse. Clearly these are important, but they also help to highlight much wider questions about sexual harassment and rights to be free from physical punishment, which might not legally be defined as abuse. A further area where young people are argued to need special protection is the circumstances under which they should work. The European Social Charter makes it clear that they should be employed only under special and restricted circumstances. Some of these restrictions are claimed because of the perceived vulnerability of new and young workers to accidents at work. The restriction of hours is argued both on grounds of health and safety and the potential impact of long or unsociable hours of work on young people's needs for education, training and social development. Below we enumerate some of these basic protection rights in turn.

(ix) Following The Children Act 1989 young people can claim:
 – **the right of protection from physical abuse.**
It is important to widen this to include:
 – **the right not to be subject to corporal punishment.**
This claim is further re-enforced by the European Convention on Human Rights.

 (x) Again following The Children Act 1989, it is clear that a young person has:
 – **the right to be free from sexual abuse.**
We wish to extend this to include:
 – **the right to be free from sexual harassment.**
Clearly, young people are protected by law from the most serious forms of sexual assault, including rape and "date rape". However, many educational institutions have now developed guidelines on sexual harassment, although little has been done yet to protect similarly the rights of young workers. As one of the most vulnerable sections of the labour market, young workers are particularly at risk. We think it is important that procedures are developed to protect young people from sexual harassment at work.

(xi) The literature on harassment and oppression suggests that young people can also suffer other forms of discrimination and abuse at school, work and in the community. They need to be protected from such abuse too. Guidelines on sexual harassment need to be paralleled by guidelines to protect the following rights:
 – **rights to protection from racial harassment;**
 – **rights to protection from harassment because of a disability;**
 – **rights to protection from harassment because of a particular form of sexuality.**

(xii) Further protection of young workers, in terms of the hours they work, and the conditions in which they do so, is more politically contentious. Following the conventions of the European Union, young people may claim:

- specific rights to health and safety at work;
- restrictions on the working hours of those under minimum school-leaving age;
- restrictions on the working hours of those undertaking education and training.

C. Representational rights

(xiii) Our discussion of representational rights (including rights to be involved in decision making) illustrated that these are of particular importance to young people in care. As with other rights which have been developed for specific groups, we argue here that it is important that representational rights should be generalizable to *all* young people:

- the rights of all young people to have an active share in decision making about their futures.

Following the Children Act 1989, we suggest that these should involve decisions about:

- education and training;
- place of abode;
- health care.

(xiv) More specifically, it is important that young people should be consulted about the running of all institutions of which they are a part. This should not only involve institutions of education, training and social care but institutions to which they are sent as a result of decisions made by the criminal justice system.

(xv) In further specifying the rights of young people to be involved in decision making about their future, we assert the "representational rights" of young people in education, in training, in place of abode, in any penal establishment in which they are confined, in health care and in employment. These rights can be further broken down into more specific claims:

- rights to read and comment on reports about them;
- rights to details about their personal background, family, or other relevant circumstances;
- rights of complaint about their treatment;
- rights of appeal against the decisions of others;
- rights to an independent external authority to hear such an appeal.

(xvi) Following the lead of the European Union on the importance of rights of representation at work, we think it important to assert the specific rights of young people at work to adequate consultation and representation in the following areas:
- the right of consultation at work on working conditions and the working environment;
- the right of consultation about the terms and conditions of training and employment.

D. Enabling rights and rights to an adequate level of resources

It was argued in Chapter 4 that it is important to see rights not only as a set of legal or moral entitlements but as closely tied to claims to resources through which they can be realized. Chapter 9, while admitting that meeting the rights of young people (claimed here) will indeed be costly, argued that this must be balanced by counting the cost of present policy failure. There are costs to the Exchequer and the community, because of failed transitions. Crime, unemployment, drop-out and failure in education and training, and homelessness, all cost dearly on the welfare budget. Most of all we wish to emphasise the human cost of failed transitions, in hopelessness, alienation, unwanted pregnancies, blighted ambitions, family conflict, a drift into crime and (the most damning of all indictments of the failure of youth policies) the escalating number of suicides committed by young people. The agenda of rights we have developed is indeed ambitious and some may argue that we cannot afford to meet it. But it is the argument of this book that we cannot afford to ignore it.

References

Abberley, P. 1992. Counting us out: a discussion of the OPCS disability surveys. *Disability Handicap and Society* 7, 139–55.

Aggleton, P., G. Hart, P. Davies 1989. *AIDS: individual, cultural and policy dimensions*. London: Falmer.

——1991. *AIDS: responses, interventions and care*. London: Falmer.

Aggleton P., H. Homans, J. Moysa, S. Watson, S. Watney 1989. *AIDS: scientific and social issues*. Edinburgh: Churchill Livingstone.

Ainley, P. 1990. *Vocational education and training*. London: Cassell.

——1991. *Young people leaving home*. London: Cassell.

Ainley, P. & M. Corney 1990. *Training for the future: the rise and fall of the Manpower Services Commission*. London: Cassell.

Allatt, P. & S. Yeandle 1992. *Youth unemployment and the family: voices of disordered times*. London: Routledge.

Allen, N. 1990. *Making sense of the Children Act*. Harlow: Longman Group UK.

Allen, S., A. Waton, K. Purcell, S. Wood 1986. *The experience of unemployment*. Basingstoke: Macmillan.

Amato, P. R. 1993a. Children's adjustment to divorce: theories, hypotheses and empirical support. *Journal of Marriage and the Family* 55, 23–38.

——1993b. Family structure, family process and family ideology. *Journal of Marriage and the Family* 55 (1), 50–54.

Anderson, I., P. Kemp, D. Quilgars 1993. *Single homeless people*. London: HMSO.

Arnot, M. & G. Weiner (eds) 1987. *Gender and the politics of schooling*. London: Hutchinson.

Ashford, S., J. Gray, M. Tanner 1993. *England and Wales Youth Cohort Study: the introduction of GCSE exams and changes in post-16 participa-

tion. Sheffield: Employment Department, Research and Development Series, Youth Cohort Series No. 23.

Ashton, D. N. 1986. *Unemployment under capitalism*. Brighton: Wheatsheaf Books.

Ashton, D. N. & D. Field 1976. *Young workers: the transition from school to work*. London: Hutchinson.

Ashton, D. N., F. Green, M. Hoskins 1989. The training system of British capitalism: changes and prospects. In *The restructuring of the British economy*, F. Green (ed.). Brighton: Harvester Wheatsheaf.

Ashton, D. N. & M. J. Maguire, with D. Bowden, P. Dellow, S. Kennedy, G. Stanley, G. Woodhead, B. Jennings 1986. *Young adults in the labour market*. London: Department of Employment, Research Paper No. 55.

Ashton, D. N., M. Maguire, M. Spilsbury 1988. Local labour markets and their impact on the life chances of youths. In *Young careers: the search for jobs and the new vocationalism*, B. Coles (ed.). Milton Keynes: Open University Press.

——1990. *Restructuring the labour market: the implications for youth*. London: Macmillan.

Ashworth, A., P. Cavadino, B. Gibson, J. Harding, A. Rutherford, P. Seago, L. Whyte 1992. *Introduction to the Criminal Justice Act 1991*. Winchester: Waterside Press.

Audit Commission–OFSTED 1993 *Unfinished business: full-time education courses for 16–19 year olds*. London: HMSO.

Bagguley, P. & K. Mann 1992. Idle, thieving bastards? Scholarly representations of the underclass. *Work, Employment and Society* 6, 113–26.

Balding, J. 1991. A study of working children in 1990. *Education and Health* 9, 4–6.

Baldwin, D. 1994. *Breaking the no job, no home cycle – hostel initiatives for young people: a case study*. BA dissertation, Department of Social Policy and Social Work, University of York.

Baldwin, S. & M. Hirst 1994. *Unequal opportunities: growing up disabled*. London: HMSO.

Baltes, P. B., D. L. Fetherstone, R. M. Lerner (eds) 1990. *Life-span development and behaviour*, vol. 10. Baum Associates.

Banks, M., I. Bates, G. Breakwell, J. Byner, N. Emler, L. Jamieson, K. Roberts 1992. *Careers and identities*. Buckingham: Open University Press.

Banks, M. & P. Ullah 1988. *Youth unemployment in the 1980s: its psychological effects*. London: Croom Helm.

Barbalet, J. M. 1988. *Citizenship*. Milton Keynes: Open University Press.

Barclay, G. C. 1993. *Digest 2; information on the criminal justice system of England and Wales*. London: Home Office.

Barn, R. 1990. Black children in local authority care: admission patterns, *New Community* 16, 229–36.

Barnes, C. 1990. *Cabbage syndrome: social construction of dependence.* Basingstoke: Falmer.

——1991. *Disabled people in Britain and discrimination.* London: Hurst & Co.

——1993. Participation and control in day centres for young disabled people aged 16 to 30 years. In *Disabling barriers – enabling environments*, J. Swain, V. Finkelstein, S. French, M. Oliver (eds). London: Sage.

Barton, L. 1986. The politics of special educational need. *Disability, Handicap and Society* 1, 273–90.

Bates, I. & G. Riseborough (eds) 1993. *Youth and inequality.* Buckingham: Open University Press.

Bauman, Z. 1992. *Intimations of postmodernity.* Cambridge: Polity Press.

Baxter, C., P. Kamaljit, L. Ward, N. Zenobia 1990. *Double discrimination: issues and services for people with learning disabilities from black and ethnic minority communities.* London: Kings Fund Centre and the Commission for Racial Equality.

Bebbington, A. & J. Miles 1989. The background of children who enter local authority care. *British Journal of Social Work* 19, 349–68.

Beck, U. 1992. *Risk society: towards a new modernity.* London: Sage.

Becker, H. 1963. *Outsiders: studies in the sociology of deviance.* New York: The Free Press.

Bell, D. 1974. *The coming of post-industrial society.* London: Heinemann Educational Books.

Bell, S. 1988. *When Salem came to the Boro.* London: Pan Books.

Bhat, A., R. Carr-Hill, S. Ohri 1988. *Britain's black population.* Aldershot: Gower.

Biehal, N., J. Clayton, M. C. Stein, J. Wade 1992. *Prepared for living.* London: National Children's Bureau.

Biggs, S. 1993. *Understanding ageing.* Buckingham: Open University Press.

Bines, W. 1993. *Homelessness and Health.* MA thesis, Department of Social Policy and Social Work, University of York.

Blaine, R. 1989. A mystery in two acts. *Special Children* 31, 5–6.

Boggan, S. 1993. Ex-convict's fight against crime founders. *The Independent*, 20 October.

Bone, M. & H. Meltzer 1989. *The prevalence of disability amongst children.* London: HMSO.

Box, S. 1987. *Recession, crime and punishment.* London: Macmillan.

Bradshaw, J. R. & J. Millar 1991. *Lone parent families.* London: Department of Social Security Research Report No. 6, HMSO.

Braid, M. 1993. Return of the bogeywoman. The *Independent on Sunday*, 10 October.

Brake, M. 1980. *The sociology of youth culture and youth subcultures.* London: Routledge & Kegan Paul.

221

Brannen, J., K. Dodd, A. Oakley, P. Storey 1994. *Young people, health and family life*. Buckingham: Open University Press.

Brewster, C. & P. Teague 1989. *European Community Social Policy; its impact on the UK*. London: Institute of Personnel Management.

Brown, P. 1987. *Schooling ordinary kids*. London: Routledge.

——1988. The new vocationalism: a policy for inequality. In *Young careers*, B. Coles (ed.), Milton Keynes: Open University Press.

Bryant, C. G. A. & D. Jary (eds) 1991. *Giddens' theory of structuration: a critical appreciation*. London: Routledge.

Bullock, R., M. Little, S. Millham 1994a. *The care careers of extremely difficult and disturbed young people: a research summary*. Dartington: Dartington Social Research Unit.

——1994b. *The experiences and careers of young people leaving youth treatment centres*. Dartington: Dartington Social Research Unit.

Burghes, L. 1993. *One-parent families: policy options for the 1990s*. York: Family Policy Studies Centre and Joseph Rowntree Foundation.

——1994. *Lone parenthood and family disruption: the outcomes for children*. London: Family Policy Studies Centre.

Burrows, R. & B. Loader (eds) 1994. *Towards a post-fordist welfare state*. London: Routledge.

Butler-Sloss, E. 1988. *Cm. 412: report of the inquiry into child abuse in Cleveland 1987*. London: HMSO.

Campbell, A. 1981. *Girl delinquents*. Oxford: Basil Blackwell.

Campbell, B. 1988. *Unofficial secrets. Child abuse: the Cleveland case*. London: Virago.

——1993. *Goliath: Britain's dangerous places*. London: Methuen.

Campbell, T. D. 1983. *The left and rights*. London: Routledge & Kegan Paul.

Carey-Wood, J., with K. Smith & P. Little 1993. *One step forward. Two steps back: providing housing for young people*. Salford: University of Salford and NCH.

Carlen, P. 1988. Out of care and into custody. In *Gender, crime and justice*, P. Carlen & A. Worrall (eds). Milton Keynes: Open University Press.

Carlen, P., D. Gleeson, J. Wardhaugh 1992. *Truancy: the politics of compulsory schooling*. Buckingham: Open University Press.

Casson, M. 1979. *Youth unemployment*. London: Macmillan.

Cavadino, M. & J. Dignan 1992. *The penal system: an introduction*. London: Sage.

Centre for Contemporary Cultural Studies (CCCS) 1981. *Unpopular education*. London: Hutchinson.

Centre for Educational Research and Innovation (CERI) 1983. *The transition from school to working life*. Paris: Organization for Economic Co-operation and Development.

——1986. *Handicapped youth at work: personal experiences of school leavers*. Paris: Organization for Economic Co-operation and Development.

——1988. *Disabled youth: the right to adult status*. Paris: Organization for Economic Co-operation and Development.

——1991. *Disabled youth: from school to work*. Paris: Organization for Economic Co-operation and Development

Chamberlaine, M. A., with S. Guthrie, M. Kettle, J. Stowe 1993. *An assessment of the health and related needs of physically handicapped young adults*. London: HMSO, Dd DH004035.

Chapman, T. & J. Cook 1989. Marginality, youth and government policy. *Critical Social Policy* **22**, 41–64.

Chase-Lansdale, P. L. & E. M. Hetherington 1990. The impact of divorce on life span development: short and long term effects. In *Life-span development and behaviour*, vol. 10, P. B. Baltes, D. L. Fetherstone, R. M. Lerner (eds). Baum Associates.

Chatrik, B. 1993. YT leavers: 1/4 unemployed; 1/3 gain qualifications. In *Working brief*. London: Unemployment Unit & Youthaid, 49.

——1994a. *Foyers: a home and a job*. London: Youthaid.

——1994b. YT guarantee: misleading official figures. In *Working brief*. London: Unemployment Unit & Youthaid, 56.

Children's Legal Centre 1984. *Working with young people*, 2nd ed. London: The Children's Legal Centre.

Chisholm, L., H. H. K. Buchner, P. Brown (eds) 1990. *Childhood, youth and social change: a comparative perspective*. Basingstoke: Falmer.

Chitty, C. & B. Simon (eds) 1993. *Education answers back: critical responses to government policy*. London: Lawrence & Wishart.

Chow, W. 1992. *An exploratory survey of detached youth work in the UK: a review and comparison with detached youth work in Hong Kong*. Unpublished MA dissertation, Department of Social Policy and Social Work, University of York.

Chubb, P. 1988. Changes in the education and training systems and implications for the work of the careers service. In *Young careers*, B. Coles (ed.). Milton Keynes: Open University Press.

Clarke, A. & M. A. Hirst 1989. Disability in adulthood: ten year follow-up of young people with disabilities. *Disability Handicap and Society* **4**, 271–83.

Cliffe, D. & D. Berridge 1991. *Closing children's homes*. London: National Children's Bureau.

Clough, E. & D. Drew 1985. *Futures in black and white*. Sheffield: Pavic Publications.

Coffield, F., C. Borrill, S. Marshall 1986. *Growing up at the margins*. Milton Keynes: Open University Press.

Cohen, N. 1993. The making of machismo. The *Independent on Sunday*, 21 October.

Cohen, S. 1980. *Folk devils and moral panics*. 2nd ed. Oxford: Martin Robertson.

Coleman J. C. & L. Hendry 1992. *The nature of adolescence*. London: Routledge.

Coleman, J. C. & C. Warren-Adamson (eds) 1992. *Youth policy in the 1990s: the way forward*. London: Routledge.

Coles, B. 1986. School leaver, job seeker, dole reeper: young and unemployed in rural England. In *The experience of unemployment*, S. Allen et al. (eds). Basingstoke: Macmillan.

Coles, B. (ed.) 1988. *Young careers: the search for jobs and the new vocationalism*. Milton Keynes: Open University Press.

Coles, B. 1991. *Partnership for prosperity*. York: NYTEC–Training Agency–Whitby Youth Trust.

——1993. *Making tracks*. York: North Yorkshire Training and Enterprise Council (NYTEC).

Coles, B. & A. J. F. Fowles 1991. *(Un)Employment, crime, offenders and their training*. Sheffield: Employment Department, Employment Services.

Coles, B. & R. F. MacDonald 1990. From new vocationalism to the culture of enterprise. In *Youth in transition*, C. Wallace & M. Cross (eds). Basingstoke: Falmer.

Coles, B. & M. Maynard 1990. Moving towards a fair start: equal opportunities and the careers service. *Gender and Education* 2, 297–308.

Commission on Social Justice 1994. *Social justice*. London: Vintage.

Confederation of British Industry (CBI) 1988. *Building a stronger partnership between business and secondary education*. London: CBI.

——1990. *The skills revolution*. London: CBI.

Connolly, M., K. Roberts, G. Ben-Tovim, P. Torkington 1992. *Black youth in Liverpool*. Culemborg, The Netherlands: Giordano Bruno.

Convery, P. & B. Chatrik 1994. 120,000 unemployed 16 & 17 year olds: 3/4 have no income. In *Working brief*. London: Unemployment Unit-Youthaid, 56.

Convery P. & D. Taylor 1994. Youth unemployment: 16 and 17 year olds. *Working brief*. London: Unemployment Unit & Youthaid, 49.

Cook, D. & B. Hudson (eds) 1993. *Racism and criminology*. London: Sage.

Coote, A. (ed.) 1992. *The welfare of citizenship: developing new social rights*. London: Institute of Public Policy Research (IPPR).

Coote, A., H. Harman, P. Hewitt 1990. *The family way: a new approach to policy making*. London: Institute for Public Policy Research (IPPR).

Corbett, J. & L. Barton 1992. *A struggle for choice: students with special needs in transition to adulthood*. London: Routledge.

Corrigan, P. 1976. Doing nothing. In *Resistance through rituals*, S. Hall & T.

Jefferson (eds). London: Hutchinson.

Courtnay, G. 1988a. *England and Wales Youth Cohort Study. Report on Cohort 1, Sweep 1*. Sheffield: Manpower Services Commission, Research and Development Series No. 41, Youth Cohort Series No. 1.

——1988b. *England and Wales Youth Cohort Study. Report on Cohort 1, Sweep 2*. Sheffield: Training Agency, Research and Development Series No. 44, Youth Cohort Series No. 3.

——1989a. *England and Wales Youth Cohort Study. Report on Cohort 3, Sweep 1*. Sheffield: Training Agency, Research and Development Series No. 53, Youth Cohort Series No. 3.

——1989b. *England and Wales Youth Cohort Study. Report on Cohort 1, Sweep 3*. Sheffield: Training Agency, Research and Development Series No. 47, Youth Cohort Series No. 4.

——1989c. *England and Wales Youth Cohort Study. Report on Cohort 2, Sweep 1*. Sheffield: Training Agency, Research and Development Series No. 48, Youth Cohort Series No. 5.

——1990a. *England and Wales Youth Cohort Study. Report on Cohort 2, Sweep 2*. Sheffield: Training Agency, Research and Development Series No. 55, Youth Cohort Series No. 9.

——1990b. *England and Wales Youth Cohort Study. Report on Cohort 2, Sweep 3*. Sheffield: Training Agency, Research and Development Series No. 59, Youth Cohort Series No. 11.

Courtnay, G., J. Gray, B. Jones, C. Pattie 1988. *England and Wales Youth Cohort Study. Routes through YTS: the experience of young people participating in the youth training scheme*. Sheffield: Manpower Services Commission, Research and Development Series No. 42, Youth Cohort Series No. 2.

Courtnay, G. & I. McAleese 1991. *England and Wales Youth Cohort Study. Report on Cohort III, Sweep 3*. Sheffield: Employment Department, Research and Development Series No. 66, Youth Cohort Series No. 17.

——1993a. *England and Wales Youth Cohort Study. Cohort IV: young people 16–17 years old in 1989, Report on Sweep 1*. Sheffield: Employment Department, Research and Development Series, Youth Cohort Series No. 21.

——1993b. *England and Wales Youth Cohort Study. Cohort 5: aged 16–17 years old in 1991, Report on Sweep 1*. Sheffield: Employment Department, Research and Development Series, Youth Cohort Series No. 22.

Craig, G. 1991. *Fit for nothing? Young people, benefits and youth training*. London: The Children's Society.

Craine, S. F. 1988. *The hoisters: survival crime and informal community networks*. Paper presented to the Group for Anthropology in Policy and Practice, 16 January 1988. University of Manchester.

——1994. *Beggars can't be choosers*. PhD thesis, Department of Sociology,

University of Salford.

Crellin E., M. L. Kellmer Pringle, P. West 1971. *Born illegitimate: a report by the National Children's Bureau*. London: National Foundation for Educational Research.

Cross, M. J., J. Wrench, S. Barnett 1990. *Ethnic minorities and the careers service*. London: Department of Employment, Research Paper No. 73.

Crow, I. 1989. *Unemployment, crime and offenders*. London: Routledge.

Dale, R. (ed.) 1985. *Education, training and employment: towards a new vocationalism?* Oxford: Pergamon.

Davies, B. 1986. *Threatening youth*. Milton Keynes: Open University Press.

Davis, T. 1994. *Young people and social security*. York: unpublished seminar paper (Department of Social Policy and Social Work).

Demo, D. H. 1993. The relentless search for effects of divorce: forging new trails or tumbling down the beaten path. *Journal of Marriage and the Family* 55, 42–5.

Dennis, N. & G. Erdos 1992. *Families without fatherhood*. Choices in Welfare Series. London: Institute of Economic Affairs, Health and Welfare Unit, No. 12.

Department for Education 1993. *Statistical bulletin, 16/93*. London: Government Statistical Service.

Department of Education and Science (DES) 1989a. *Report by HMI inspectors on a survey of provision for pupils with emotional/behavioural difficulties in maintained special schools and unit*. London: DES.

——1989b. *Report by HMI inspectors on educating physically disabled pupils*. London: DES.

——1989c. *Report by HMI inspectors on the effectiveness of small special schools*. London: DES.

——1991. *Technical and Vocational Education Initiative (TVEI): England and Wales 1983–90*. London: HMSO.

Department of Education and Science, Department of Employment, Welsh Office 1991. *Education and training for the 21st century*. White Paper Cm. 1536. London: HMSO.

Department of Employment 1988. *Employment in the 1990s*. Cm. 540. London: HMSO.

Department of Health 1991. *The Children Act 1989. Guidance and regulations:* vols 1–9. London: HMSO.

——1992. *Health and personal social services statistics for England*. London: HMSO.

——1993. *Report on the implementation of the children act 1989*. London: HMSO.

DHSS 1985. *Review of child care law: report to ministers of an inter-departmental working party*. London: HMSO.

——1987. *The law on child care and family services*. Cm. 62. London:

HMSO.

Ditchfield, J. & L. Catan 1992. *Juveniles sentenced for serious offences: a comparison of regimes in young offender institutions and local authority community homes.* London: Home Office Research and Planning Paper No. 66.

Doyal, L. & I. Gough 1984. A theory of human need. *Critical Social Policy* 10, 6–38.

——1991. *A theory of human need.* London: Macmillan.

Drew, D. & J. Gray 1991. The black and white gap in examination results. *New Community* 17, 159–72.

Elliott, B. J. & M. P. M. Richards 1991a. Children and divorce: educational performance and behaviour before and after parental separation. *International Journal of Law and the Family* 5, 258–76.

——1991b. Parental divorce and the life chances of children. *Family Law*, November, 481–4.

Employment Department 1992. *The United Kingdom in Europe: people, jobs and progress.* London: Employment Department.

Employment Gazette 1988. Ethnic origins and the labour market, December, 633–46.

Farrington, D. P. 1990. Implications of criminal career research for the prevention of offending. *Journal of Adolescence* 13, 93–113.

——1992. Trends in English juvenile delinquency and their explanations. *International Journal of Comparative and Applied Criminal Justice* 16, 151–63.

Featherstone, M. 1990. Global culture: an introduction. *Theory, Culture and Society* 7, 1–14.

Felstead, A. & F. Green 1993. *Cycles of training? Evidence from the British recession of the early 1990s.* Leicester: University of Leicester, Department of Economics, Discussion Paper in Economics, 93/3.

Fenton, M. & P. Hughes 1989. *Passivity to empowerment: a living skills curriculum for people with disabilities.* London: Royal Association for Disability and Rehabilitation.

Ferguson, T. & A. Kerr 1960. *Handicapped youth.* Oxford: Oxford University Press.

Ferri, E. 1984. *Step children: a national study.* London, NFER-Nelson.

Field, F. 1990. *Losing out: the emergence of Britain's underclass.* Oxford: Blackwell.

——1993. *An agenda for Britain.* London: Harper Collins.

Finch, J. 1989. *Family obligation and social change.* Cambridge: Polity Press.

Finch, J. & J. Mason 1993. *Negotiating family responsibilities.* London: Routledge.

Finn, D. 1987. *Training without jobs.* Basingstoke: Macmillan.

First Key 1987. *A study of young black people leaving care*. Leeds: First Key.

Fish, J. 1986. *Young people with handicaps: the road to adulthood*. Paris: Centre for Education Research and Innovation, OECD.

Flynn, M. & M. Hirst 1992. *This year, next year, sometime . . .? Learning disability and adulthood*. London and York: National Development Team, Social Policy Research Unit, University of York.

Foster, J. 1990. *Villains*. London: Routledge.

Fox-Harding, L. 1991. *Perspectives in child care policy*. London: Longman.

Franklin, B. (ed.) 1986. *The rights of children*. Oxford: Basil Blackwell.

Fraser, D. 1984. *The evolution of the welfare state*. London: Macmillan.

Freeman, M. D. A. 1983. *The rights and wrongs of children*. London: Frances Pinter.

Frost, N. & M. Stein 1989. *The politics of child welfare*. Hemel Hempstead: Harvester Wheatsheaf.

Fry, E. 1992. *After care: making the most of foster care*. London: National Foster Care Association.

Fryer, D. 1992. Psychological or material deprivation: why does unemployment have mental health consequences? In *Understanding unemployment*, E. McLaughlin. London: Routledge.

Fulcher, G. (ed.) 1989. *Disabling policies? A comparative approach to education policy and disability*. London: Falmer.

Furlong, A. 1992. *Growing up in a classless society? School to work transitions*. Edinburgh: Edinburgh University Press.

Furlong, A. & G. H. Cooney 1990. Getting on their bikes: teenagers leaving home in Scotland in the 1980s. *Journal of Social Policy* 19, 535–51.

Gallie, D., C. March, C. Vogler 1993. *Social change and the experience of unemployment*. Oxford: Oxford University Press.

Garnett, L. 1992. *Leaving care and after*. London: National Children's Bureau.

Gelsthorpe, L. & A. Morris 1994. Juvenile justice 1945–1992. In *The Oxford Handbook of Criminology*, M. Maguire, M. Morgan, R. Reiner (eds). Oxford: Clarendon Press.

General Household Survey 1989. London: HMSO.

Giddens, A. 1976. *New rules of sociological method: a positive critique of interpretive sociologies*. London: Hutchinson.

——1979. *Central problems in social theory*. Basingstoke: Macmillan.

——1982. *Profiles and critiques in social theory*. London: Macmillan.

——1991. Structuration theory: past, present and future. In *Giddens' theory of structuration: a critical appreciation*, C. G. A. Bryant & D. Jary (eds). London: Routledge.

Gilder, G. 1982. *Wealth and poverty*. London: Buchan & Enright.

——1986. *Men and marriage*. Gretna, Louisiana: Penguin.

——1987. The collapse of the American family. *The Public Interest* 89,

20–5.

Gleeson, D. (ed.) 1983. *Youth training and the search for work*. London: Routledge & Kegan Paul.

Gleeson, D. 1989. *The paradox of training*. Milton Keynes: Open University Press.

Glendinning, C. & J. Millar (eds) 1987. *Women and poverty in Britain*. Brighton: Wheatsheaf Books.

Gottesmann, M. 1994. *Recent changes and new trends in extra-familial child care: an international perspective*. London: Whiting & Birch.

Graham, J. 1988. *Schools, disruptive behaviours and delinquency*. London: HMSO, Home Office Research Study No. 96.

Gray, J., D. Jesson, C. Pattie, N. Sime 1989. *England and Wales Youth Cohort Study. Education and training opportunities in the inner city*. Sheffield: Training Agency, Research and Development Series No. 51, Youth Cohort Series No. 7.

Gray, J., D. Jesson, M. Tranmer 1993. *England and Wales Youth Cohort Study. Boosting post-16 participation in full-time education: a study of some key factors*. Sheffield: Employment Department, Research and Development Series, Youth Cohort Series No. 20.

Gray, J. & N. Sime 1990. *England and Wales Youth Cohort Study. Patterns of participation in full-time post-compulsory education*. Sheffield: Training Agency, Research and Development Series No. 61, Youth Cohort Series No 13.

Green, F. (ed.) 1989. *The restructuring of the British economy*. Brighton: Harvester Wheatsheaf.

Griffin, C. 1985. *Typical girls: young women from school to the job market*. London: Routledge & Kegan Paul.

Hall, C., S. Chritcher, T. Jefferson, J. Clarke, B. Roberts 1978. *Policing the crisis*. London: Macmillan.

Hall, S. & T. Jefferson (eds) 1976. *Resistance through ritual*. London: Hutchinson.

Halsey, A. H. 1991. Time to rebuild the traditional family. London: *Financial Times*.

——1992. Foreword. In *Families without fatherhood*, N. Dennis & G. Erdos. London: IEA, Health and Welfare Unit, No. 12.

Hansard 21 March 1985: col. 1004–5.

Harris, N. S. 1989. *Social security for young people*. Aldershot: Avebury.

——1990. Social security and the transition to adulthood. *Journal of Social Policy* 19, 501–23.

Harris, R. J. & D. Webb 1987. *Welfare, power, and juvenile justice*. London: Tavistock.

Harvey, D. 1989. *The condition of postmodernity*. London: Blackwells.

Haskey, J. 1990. Children in families broken by divorce. *Population Trends*

61, 34–62.

——1991. Estimated numbers and demographic characteristics of one-parent families in Great Britain. *Population Trends* 65, 35–47.

——1992. Pre-marital cohabitation and the probability of subsequent divorce: an analysis using new data from the GHS. *Population Trends* 68 34–62.

——1993. Trends in the number of one-parent families in Great Britain. *Population Trends* 71, 26–33.

——1994. Stepfamilies and stepchildren in Great Britain. *Population Trends* 76, 17–28.

Haviland, J. (ed.) 1988. *Take care Mr. Baker*. London: Fourth Estate.

Heath, A., M. Colton, J. Aldgate 1989. Educational progress of children in and out of care. *British Journal of Social Work* 19, 447–60.

Hebdige, D. 1979. *Subcultures: the meaning of style*. London: Methuen.

——1988. *Hiding in the light*. London: Routledge.

Heddy, J. 1991. *Housing for young people*. Paris: Union des Foyers des Jeunes Travailleurs (UFJT).

Hendry, L. B. 1983. *Growing up and going out*. Aberdeen: Aberdeen University Press.

Hills, J. (ed.) 1991. *The state of welfare: the welfare state in Britain since 1974*. Oxford: Clarendon.

Hirst, M. A. 1983. Young people with disabilities: what happens after 16. *Child Care Health and Development* 9, 273–84.

——1985a. Social security and insecurity. *International Social Security Review* 85, 258–72.

——1985b. Could schools do more for leavers? *British Journal of Special Education* 12, 143–6.

——1987. Careers of young people with disabilities between the ages of 15 and 21 years. *Disability, Handicap and Society* 2, 61–74.

——1991. *National survey of young people with disabilities*. York: Social Policy Research Unit.

Hollands, R. G. 1990. *The long transition: class, culture and youth training*. Basingstoke: Macmillan.

Hollands, R. 1991. Youth training for post industrialism. *Youth and Policy*, 9–19.

Home Office 1990. *Crime, justice and protecting the public*. Cm. 965. London: HMSO.

Home Office Research and Statistics Department 1989. *Bulletin: criminal careers of those born in 1953 and 1963*. London: Home Office, 27/89.

——1993. *Bulletin*. London: Home Office, 9/93.

——1993. *Digest 2: information on the criminal justice system in England and Wales*, London: Home Office.

Hough, M. & P. Mayhew 1983. *The British crime survey: first report*. London: HMSO, Home Office Research Study No. 85.

House of Commons, Home Affairs Committee 1993. *Sixth report: juvenile offenders, volume 1*. London: HMSO.

Howard League for Penal Reform 1993a. *Dying in prison*. London: Howard League for Penal Reform.

——1993b. *Young and in trouble: young teenagers and crime*. London: Howard League for Penal Reform.

Hughes, J. M. (ed.) 1984. *The best years: reflections of school leavers in the 1980s*. Aberdeen: Aberdeen University Press.

Hutson, S. & R. Jenkins 1987. *Taking the strain: families, unemployment and the transition to adulthood*. Milton Keynes: Open University Press.

Hutson, S. & M. Liddiard 1991. *Young and homeless in Wales*. Swansea: Department of Sociology and Anthropology, University College, Swansea.

Inspectorate of Schools 1991. *Technical and Vocational Educational Initiative (TVEI) England and Wales 1983–90*. London: HMSO.

Institute of Economic Affairs 1990. *The emerging British underclass*. London: Institute of Economic Affairs, Health and Welfare Unit.

Jackson, S. 1988a. The education of children in care, *Bristol Papers No. 1*. Bristol School of Applied Social Services, University of Bristol.

——1988b. Residential care and education. *Children and Society* 4, 335–50.

Jahoda, M. 1982. *Employment and unemployment: a socio–psychological analysis*. Cambridge: Cambridge University Press.

Jeffs, T. & M. Smith (eds) 1988. *Welfare and youth work practice*. Basingstoke: Macmillan.

Jenkins, R. 1983. *Lads, citizens and ordinary kids*. London: Routledge & Kegan Paul.

Jesson, D. & J. Gray 1990. *England and Wales Youth Cohort Study. Access, entry and potential demand for higher education amongst 18–19 year olds in England and Wales*. Sheffield: Training Agency, Research and Development Series No. 60, Youth Cohort Series No. 12.

Jesson, D., J. Gray, N. Sime 1991. *England and Wales Youth Cohort Study. Participation, progress and performance in post-compulsory education*. Sheffield: Employment Department, Research and Development Series No. 64, Youth Cohort Series No. 15.

Jessop, B. 1988. Regulation theory, post-Fordism and the state. *Capital and Class* 34, 146–68.

Jewson, N. & D. Mason 1986. The theory and practice of equal opportunities policies: liberal and radical approaches. *Sociological Review* 34, 307–34.

Jones, B., J. Gray, E. Clough 1988. Finding a post-16 route – the first year's experience. In *Young careers: the search for jobs and the new vocationalism*, B. Coles (ed.). Milton Keynes: Open University Press.

Jones, G. 1987. Leaving the parental home; an analysis of early housing careers. *Journal of Social Policy* **16**, 49–74.

——1991. The cost of living in the parental home. *Youth and Policy* **32**, 19–29.

——1993a. *Regulated entry into the housing market? the process of leaving home*, Young People in and out of the Housing Market, Working Paper 2. Edinburgh: Centre for Educational Sociology, University of Edinburgh.

——1993b. *On the margins of the housing market: housing and homelessness in youth*, Young People in and out of the Housing Market, Working Paper 3. Edinburgh: Centre for Educational Sociology, University of Edinburgh.

——1994. *Family support for young people: a research report*. Edinburgh: Centre for Educational Sociology, University of Edinburgh.

Jones, G. & L. Gilliland 1993. *"I would hate to be young again": biographies of risk and its avoidance*, Young People in and out of the Housing Market. Working Paper 4. Edinburgh: Centre for Educational Sociology, University of Edinburgh.

Jones, G. & C. Wallace 1992. *Youth family and citizenship*. Milton Keynes: Open University Press.

Kelly, B. 1992. *Children inside – rhetoric and practice in a locked institution for children*. London: Routledge.

Kiernan, K. 1992. The impact of family disruption in childhood on transitions made in young adult life. *Population Studies* **46**, 213–34.

Kiernan, K. & M. Wicks 1990. *Family change and future policy*. York: Joseph Rowntree Memorial Trust–Family Policy Studies Centre.

Killeen, J., M. White, A. G. Watts 1992. *The economic value of careers guidance*. London: Policy Studies Institute–National Institute for Careers Education and Counselling.

Kirk, D., S. Nelson, A. Sinfield, D. Sinfield 1991. *Excluding youth: poverty among young people living away from home*. Edinburgh: Bridges Project, Edinburgh Centre for Social Welfare Research, Department of Social Policy and Social Work, University of Edinburgh.

Kolvin, I., F. J. W. Millar, D. Scott, S. R. M. Gatzanis, M. Fleeting 1990. *Continuities of deprivation*, ESRC/DHSS studies in deprivation and disadvantage. Aldershot: Avebury.

Kuh, D. & M. Maclean 1990. Women's childhood experience of parental separation and their subsequent health and status in adulthood. *Journal of Biosocial Science* **22**, 121–35.

Lash, S. 1990. *Sociology of postmodernism*. London: Routledge.

Lavalette, M. 1994. *Child employment in the capitalist labour market*. Aldershot: Avebury.

Lavalette, M., S. Hobbs, J. McKechnie 1995 (forthcoming). Child employment in Britain. *Youth and Policy*.

Lee, D., D. Marsden, P. Rickman, J. Duncombe 1990. *Scheming for youth: a study of YTS in the enterprise culture.* Milton Keynes: Open University Press.

Lee, D. J. 1990. Surrogate employment, surrogate labour markets and the development of youth training policies in the eighties. In *Youth in transition*, C. Wallace & M. Cross (eds). Basingstoke: Falmer.

Lees, S. & J. Mellor 1986. Girls' rights. In *The rights of children*, R. A. Franklin (ed.). Oxford: Basil Blackwell.

Leonard, M. 1988. *The education act: a tactical guide for schools.* Oxford: Blackwell Education.

Levy, A. & B. Kahan 1991. *The pindown experience* (The Report of the Staffordshire Child Care Inquiry 1990). Stafford: Staffordshire County Council.

Liddiard, M. & S. Hutson 1991. Youth homelessness in Wales. In *Youth in transition*, C. Wallace & M. Cross (eds). Basingstoke: Falmer.

Lister, R. 1990. Women, economic dependency and citizenship. *Journal of Social Policy* 19, 445–67.

——1991. *The exclusive society: citizenship and the poor.* London: Child Poverty Action Group.

Little, M. 1990. *Young men in prison.* Aldershot: Dartmouth Publishing Company.

Lunt, N. & P. Thornton 1993. *Employment policies for disabled people: a review of legislation and services in fifteen countries.* Sheffield: Employment Department, Research Series No. 16.

Mac an Ghaill, M. 1988. *Young, gifted and black.* Milton Keynes, Open University Press.

MacDonald, R. F. 1988. Out of town, out of work: research on post-sixteen experience in two rural areas. In *Young careers*, B. Coles (ed.). Milton Keynes: Open University Press.

——1994. Fiddly jobs, undeclared working and the "something for nothing society". *Work, Employment and Society* 8, 507–30.

Maclagan, I. 1993. Youth wages drop. In *Working brief.* London: Unemployment Unit & Youthaid, 49.

McLaughlin, E. (ed.) 1992. *Understanding employment.* London: Routledge.

McLaughlin, E. 1994. *Flexibility in work and benefits.* London: IPPR.

Maclean, M. & M. E. J. Wadsworth 1988. The interests of children after parental divorce: a long-term perspective. *International Journal of Law and the Family* 2, 155–66.

Maclure, J. S. 1988. *Education re-formed: a guide to the Education Act 1988.* London: Hodder & Stoughton.

Maguire, M., M. Morgan, R. Reiner (eds) 1994. *The Oxford handbook of criminology.* Oxford: Clarendon Press.

233

Major, J. 1993. Speech to the 1993 Conservative Party Conference at Black-pool. Text reported in the *Guardian*, 9 October.

Makeham, P. 1980. *Youth unemployment: an examination of evidence on youth unemployment using national statistics*. London: Department of Employment, Research Paper No. 10.

Mann, K. 1992. *The making of an English underclass?* Buckingham: Open University Press.

Mann, P. 1987. Ruling class strategy and citizenship. *Sociology* 21. 339–54.

Manpower Services Commission 1977. *Young people and work* (The Holland Report). London: Manpower Services Commission.

——1981. *A new training initiative*. London: Manpower Services Commission.

Marsh, P., E. Rosser, R. Harre 1978. *The rules of disorder*. London: Routledge & Kegan Paul.

Marshall, T. H. 1963. Citizenship and social class. In *Sociology at the cross roads*, T. H. Marshall. London: Heinemann.

——1981. *The right to welfare*. London: Heinemann.

Martin, J., H. Meltzer, D. Elliot 1988. *The prevalence of disability among adults*. London: HMSO.

Mayhew, N., C. Mierall-Black, N. Maung 1993. *The 1992 British crime survey*. London: HMSO, Home Office Research Study.

Mead, L. 1986. *Beyond entitlement: the social obligations of citizenship*. New York: Free Press.

Meltzer, H., N. Robus, M. Smyth 1989. *Disabled children: services, transport and education*. London: HMSO.

MENCAP 1993. *Pathway employment service: report 1992–3*. York: MENCAP.

Merchant, J. & R. MacDonald 1994. Youth and the rave culture, ecstasy and health. *Youth and Policy* 45, 16–38.

Metcalf, H. 1992. Hidden unemployment and the labour market. In *Understanding unemployment*, E. McLaughlin (ed.). London: Routledge.

Mirza, H. S. 1992. *Young, female and black*. London: Routledge.

Mitzen, P. 1993. Youth training: consensus or conflict in the 1990s. *Youth and Policy* 43, 36–43.

Morgan, S. & P. Righton (eds) 1989. *Child care: concerns and conflicts*. London: Hodder & Stoughton.

Morris, L. 1994. *Dangerous classes: the underclass and social citizenship*. London: Routledge.

Morris, P. 1992. Too much too young. *Social Work Today* 24 (8 October), 18–19.

Muncie, J. 1984. *The trouble with kids today*. London: Hutchinson.

Murray, C. 1984. *Loosing ground*. New York: Basic Books.

——1990. *The emerging British underclass*. London: Institute of Economic

Affairs.

Myrdal, G. 1962. *Challenge to affluence*. London: Victor Gollancz.

NACRO 1989. *Progress through partnership: the role of statutory and voluntary agencies in the funding and management of schemes for juvenile offenders established under the DHSS Intermediate Treatment Initiative.* London: NACRO.

——1991a. *Black people's experience of criminal justice*. London: NACRO.

——1991b. *Seizing the initiative: NACRO's final report on the DHSS intermediate treatment initiative to divert juvenile offenders from care and custody: 1983–89*. London: NACRO.

——1993. *Community provision for young people in the youth justice system*. London: NACRO.

National Association of Citizens Advice Bureau (NACAB) 1989. *Income support for 16–17-year-olds*. London: NACAB.

National Association of Citizens Advice Bureau (NACAB) 1992. *Severe hardship payments; CAB evidence of young people's benefits*. London: NACAB.

National Council for Vocational Qualifications (NCVC) 1993. A Statement by the National Council for Vocational Qualifications on *All our futures – Britain's education revolution*. London: Channel Four Television.

National Children's Home (NCH) 1993. *A lost generation?* London: NCH.

National Curriculum Council (NCC) 1991. *Work experience and the school curriculum*. York: NCC.

National Foster Care Association (NFCA) 1992. *After care: making the most of foster care*. London: NFCA.

Newman, C. 1989. *Young runaways: findings from Britain's first safe house*. London: Children's Society.

Noller, P. & V. Callan 1991. *The adolescent in the family*. London: Routledge.

Novak, M. 1987. Welfare's "New Consensus": Reply to Gilder. *The Public Interest* 89, 26–30.

OFSTED 1993. *GNVQs in schools: the introduction of general national vocational qualifications 1992*. London: HMSO.

Oliver, M. 1990. *The politics of disablement*. Houndmills: Macmillan.

——1993. Re-defining disability: a challenge to research. In *Disabling barriers – enabling environments*. J. Swain, V. Finkelstein, S. French, M. Oliver (eds). London: Sage.

Parker, G. 1984. *Into work: a review of the literature about disabled young adults' preparation for and movement into work*. York: Social Policy Research Unit, University of York.

Parker, H., M. Casburn, D. Turnball 1981. *Receiving juvenile justice*. Oxford: Blackwells.

Parsons, T. 1942. Age and sex in the social structure of the United States. Reprinted in Parsons, T. 1954. *Essays in sociological theory*. New York:

The Free Press.

Parton, N. 1991. *Governing the family: child protection and the state*. London: Macmillan.

Pearson, G. 1983. *Hooligan: a history of respectable fears*. Basingstoke: Macmillan.

Phillips, A. 1993. *The trouble with boys*. London: Pandora.

Pissarides, C. & J. Wadsworth 1992. Unemployment risks. In *Understanding unemployment*, E. McLaughlin (ed.). London: Routledge.

Pitts, J. 1988. *The politics of juvenile crime*. London: Sage.

——1993. Theorotyping: anti-racism, criminology and black young people. In *Racism and criminology*, D. Cook & B. Hudson (eds). London: Sage.

Plant, M. & M. Plant 1992. *Risk takers: alcohol, drugs, sex and youth*. London: Routledge.

Plant, R. 1988. *Citizenship, rights and socialism*. London: Fabian Society.

Popay, J. & G. Jones 1990. Patterns of health and illness amongst lone parents. *Journal of Social Policy* **19**, 499–534.

Pritchard, J. 1982. *The Penguin guide to the law*. London: Penguin.

Quilgars, D. & I. Anderson 1993. Housing, jobs, and the welfare of young people: what foyers can achieve. In *Housing and welfare*, P. Malpass & A. Baines (eds) Bristol: SAUS, Housing Studies Association Proceedings.

Raffe, D. 1986. The context of the Youth Training Scheme: an analysis of its strategy and development. Edinburgh: Centre for Educational Sociology, University of Edinburgh, Working Paper No. 8611.

Raffe, D. (ed.) 1988. *Education and the youth labour market*. Lewes: Falmer.

Randall, G. 1988. *No way home*. London: Centrepoint.

——1989. *Homeless and hungry*. London: Centrepoint.

Rees, T. L. & P. Atkinson (eds) 1982. *Youth unemployment and state intervention*. London: Routledge & Kegan Paul.

Regional Trends 1994. Table 4.5, 55. London: HMSO.

Reiser, R. & M. Mason 1990. *Disability equality in the classroom: a human rights issue*. London: Inner London Education Authority.

Richardson, S. A. 1978. Careers of mentally retarded young persons; services, jobs, and interpersonal relations. *American Journal of Mental Deficiency* **82**, 349–58.

Rickford, F. 1992. Moving on. *Social Work Today* **24** (24 September), 16–18.

Ritzer, G. 1993. *The McDonaldization of society*. New York: Pine Forge.

Roberts, D. J. 1975. A survey of 235 Salford handicapped school leavers for 1970–72. *Public Health* **89**, 207–11.

Roberts, K. 1984. *School leavers and their prospects; youth and the labour market in the 1980s*. Milton Keynes: Open University Press.

——1993. Career trajectories and the mirage of increased social mobility. In

Youth and Inequality, I. Bates & G. Riseborough (eds). Buckingham: Open University Press.

Roberts, K. & C. Chadwick 1991. *England and Wales Youth Cohort Study. Transitions into the labour market: new routes of the 1980s. A study of transitions 1984–87.* Sheffield: Employment Department, Research and Development Series No. 65, Youth Cohort Series No. 16.

Roberts, K., S. Dench, D. Richardson 1986. Firms' uses of the Youth Training Scheme, *Policy Studies* 6, 37–53.

Roberts, K., S. Dench, D. Richardson 1987. *The changing structure of the youth labour market.* London: Department of Employment, Research Paper No. 59.

Robertson, R. 1990. Mapping the global condition: globilization as the central concept. *Theory Culture and Society* 7, 15–30.

Robins, D. 1992. *Tarnished vision: crime and conflict in the inner city.* Oxford: Oxford University Press.

Roche, M. 1987. Citizenship, social theory and social change. *Theory and Society* 16, 363–99.

———1992. *Re-thinking citizenship: welfare, ideology and change in modern society.* Cambridge: Polity Press.

Rodgers, R. 1986. *Caught in the act.* London: Centre for Studies in the Integration in Education–the Spastics Society.

Roll, J. 1990. *Young people: growing up in the welfare state.* London: Family Policy Studies Centre.

Rowe, J., M. Hundleby, L. Garnett 1989. *Child care now.* London: British Agency for Adoption and Fostering (BAAF).

Rutherford, A. 1986. *Growing out of crime.* Harmondsworth: Penguin.

———1992. *Growing out of crime.* Winchester: Waterside Press.

Rutter, M., B. Maughan, P. Mortimore, P. Ouston, A. Smith 1979 *Fifteen thousand hours.* London: Open Books.

Rutter, M. & H. Giller 1983. *Juvenile delinquency: trends and perspectives.* Harmondsworth: Penguin.

Saddington, A. 1991. Something is going dramatically wrong. *Community Care*, 3 October.

Schweinhart, L. J. & D. Weikhart 1993. *A summary of the significant benefits of the High/Scope Perry preschool study through age 27.* Ypsilanti, Michigan: High/Scope Press.

Segal, S. & V. Varma (eds) 1991. *Prospects for people with learning difficulties.* London: David Fulton.

Sillitoe, K. & H. Meltzer 1985. *The West Indian school leaver: Vol. 1, Starting work.* OPCS, Social Survey Division. London: HMSO.

Sime, N. 1991. *England and Wales Youth Cohort Study. Constraining choices: unemployment amongst sixteen and seventeen year olds in the late eighties.* Sheffield: Employment Department, Research and Development

Series No. 67, Youth Cohort Series No. 18.

Sime, N., C. Pattie, J. Gray 1990. *England and Wales Youth Cohort Study. What now? The transition from school to the labour market amongst 16 to 19 year olds.* Sheffield: Training Agency, Research and Development Series No. 62, Youth Cohort Series No. 14.

Simon, B. 1988. *Bending the rules: the Baker reform of education.* London: Lawrence & Wishart.

Simon, F. & I. Crow 1990. *Training young offenders.* London: NACRO.

Simpson, P. 1990. Education for disabled children – today and tomorrow. *Contact* 64, 9–11.

Skeggs, B. 1986. *Young women and further education: a case study of young women's experience of caring courses in a local college.* Unpublished PhD thesis, Department of Education, University of Keele.

Skeggs, B. 1990. Gender reproduction and further education: domestic apprenticeships. In *Training and its alternatives*, D. Gleeson (ed.). Milton Keynes: Open University Press.

Skellington, R., P. Morris, P. Gordon 1992. *"Race" in Britain today.* London: Sage and Open University Press.

Sly, F. 1993. Economic activity of 16 and 17 year olds. *Employment Gazette,* July.

Smart, B. 1993. *Postmodernity.* London: Routledge.

Smith, D. J. (ed.) 1992. *Understanding the underclass.* London: Policy Studies Institute.

Smith, M. 1988. *Developing youth work.* Milton Keynes: Open University Press.

Smithers, A. 1993. *All our futures: Britain's education revolution.* London: Channel Four Television.

Smyth, M. & N. Robus 1989. *The financial circumstances of families with disabled children living in private households.* London: OPCS.

Social Services Committee (HC 360) 1984. *Children in care.* London: HMSO.

Social Services Inspectorate 1994. *Responding to youth crime: findings from inspections of youth justice services in five local authority social service departments.* London: HMSO.

Solomos, J. 1988. *Black youth, racism and the state.* Cambridge: Cambridge University Press.

——1993. Constructions of black criminality: racialisation and criminalisation in perspective. In *Racism and criminology*, D. Cook & B. Hudson (eds). London: Sage.

Standing, G. 1986. *Unemployment and the labour market: the UK.* Geneva: International Labour Office.

Stein, M. 1991. *Leaving care and the 1989 Children Act, the agenda.* Leeds: First Key.

Stein, M. & M. Carey 1986 *Leaving care*. Oxford: Basil Blackwell

Stone, M. 1989. *Young people leaving care*. London: The Royal Philanthropic Society.

Stowell, R. 1987. *Catching up?* London: National Bureau for Handicapped Students (now SKILL: National Bureau for Students with Disability).

Swain, J., V. Finkelstein, S. French, M. Oliver 1993. *Disabling barriers – enabling environments*. London: Sage.

Swann, W. 1988. Trends in special school placements to 1986: measuring, assessing and explaining segregation. *Oxford Review of Education* **14**, 139–61.

Sykes, G. M. & D. Matza 1957. Techniques of neutralization: a theory of delinquency. *American Sociological Review* **22**, 664–70.

Tarling, R. 1993. *Analysing offending*. London: HMSO.

Taylor, D. 1993. Exchequer costs of unemployment. In *Working Brief*. London: Unemployment Unit & Youthaid, 49.

Taylor, L. 1971. *Deviance and Society*. London: Nelson.

——1984. *In the underworld*. Oxford: Blackwell.

Thornton, R. 1990. *The new homeless: the crisis of youth homelessness and the response of local housing authorities*. London: SHAC.

Thorpe, R. 1974. Mum and Mrs So and So. *Social Work Today* **22**, 694.

Tomlinson, S. 1982. *The sociology of special education*. London: Routledge & Kegan Paul.

——1990. Report: education and training. *New Community* **19**, 97–104.

Triseloitis, J. 1980. *New developments in foster care and adoption*. London: Routledge & Kegan Paul.

Troyna, B. & D. I. Smith 1983. *Racism, school and the labour market*. Leicester: National Youth Bureau.

Tuck, M. 1993. Quoted in D. Hare. Your fears are exaggerated. *Independent* (10 October 1993).

Turner, B. 1986. *Citizenship and capitalism*. London: Allen & Unwin.

——1990. Outline of a theory of citizenship. *Sociology* **24**, 189–217.

Ullah, P. 1985. Disaffected black and white youth: the role of unemployment duration and perceived job discrimination. *Ethnic and Racial Studies* **8**, 2.

——1987. Unemployed black youths in a northern city. In *Unemployed people*, D. Fryer & P. Ullah (eds). Milton Keynes: Open University Press.

University Grants Committee (UGC) 1989. *Report of the review committee on social policy and administration*. London: UGC.

Utting, D., J. Bright, C. Henricson 1993. *Crime and the family*. London: Family Policy Study Centre.

Utting, W. B. 1991. *Children in the public care* (The Utting Report). London: HMSO.

Verma, G. K. & C. Bagley (eds) 1979. *Race, education and identity*. London:

Macmillan.

Verma, G. K. & D. S. Darby 1987. *Race, training and employment*. Lewes: Falmer.

Wadsworth, M. 1979. *The roots of delinquency*, London: Martin Robertson.

Wadsworth, M. E. J. & M. Maclean 1986. Parents' divorce and children's life chances. *Children and Youth Services Review* 8.

Wagner, N. 1992. *Choosing With care* (The Report of the Committee of Inquiry into the Selection, Development and Management of Staff in Children's Homes). London: HMSO.

Walby, S. 1994. Is citizenship gendered? *Sociology* **28**, 379–95.

Walker, A. 1982. *Unqualified and underemployed*. Basingstoke: Macmillan and National Children's Bureau.

Walker, R. 1991. *Thinking about workfare*. London: HMSO.

Walker, S. & L. Barton (eds). 1986. *Youth unemployment and schooling*. Milton Keynes: Open University Press.

Wallace, C. 1987. *For richer for poorer: growing up in and out of work*. London: Tavistock Publications Limited.

Wallace, C. & M. Cross (eds) 1990. *Youth in transition*. Basingstoke: Falmer.

Walmsley, R., L. Howard, S. White 1992. *The National Prison Survey 1991: main findings*. London: Home Office Research Study No. 128.

Ward, K., S. Riddell, M. Dyer, G. Thompson 1991. *The transition to adulthood of young people with recorded special educational needs*. Stirling and Edinburgh: Departments of Education, University of Edinburgh and University of Stirling.

Warnock, M. W. 1978. *Special educational needs: report of the committee of enquiry into the education of handicapped children and young people*. Cmnd. 7212. London: HMSO.

White, R. & D. Brockington 1983. *Tales out of school*. London: Routledge & Kegan Paul.

White, R., P. Carr, N. Lowe 1990. *A guide to the Children Act 1989*. London: Butterworths.

Whitfield, K. & C. Bourlakis 1990. *England and Wales Youth Cohort Study. YTS and the labour queue*. Sheffield: Training Agency, Research and Development Series No. 54, Youth Cohort Series No. 8.

Williams, G. & D. McCreadie 1992. *Ty Mawr Community Home inquiry*. Swansea: Gwent County Council.

Williamson, H. 1993. Youth policy in the United Kingdom and the marginalisation of young people. *Youth and Policy* **40**, 33–48.

Willis, P. 1977. *Learning to labour*. Farnborough: Saxon House.

——1984. Youth unemployment. *New Society*, 29 March, 5 April, 12 April.

Wilson, H. 1975. Juvenile delinquency, parental criminality and social handicap. *British Journal of Criminology* **20**, 203–35.

Wilson, J. Q. & R. J. Hernstein 1985. *Crime and human nature*. New York: Touchstone and Simon and Schuster.

Woodroffe, C. M. Glickman, M. Barker, C. Power 1993. *Children, teenagers and health: the key data*. Buckingham: Open University Press.

Wright, M. 1988. *Young people's rights*. London: Optima books.

——1990. *Young people's rights*. London: MacDonald Optima.

Young, P. 1985. *Mastering social welfare*. London: Macmillan.

Zaretsky, E. 1976. *Capitalism, family and personal life*. London: Pluto.

Author index

Subject index